REDISCOVERING
MY BODY

Rediscovering My Body
1st Edition
The Galeano Group
thegaleanogroup.com
2525 Araphoe Ave
Suite E4, pmb-324
Boulder, CO. 80302

Set in Garamond and Benguiat
Title set in Orpheus Pro
Illustrations: Cat Yoon
Design: A. Kierson
Photography: Anthony Camera
Copyright © 2020 by Tara Galeano

The information contained in this book is intended to be
educational and not for diagnosis, prescription, or treatment
of any health disorder whatsoever. This information should
not replace consultation with a competent healthcare
professional. The content of this book is intended to
be used as an adjunct to a rational and responsible
healthcare program prescribed by a professional healthcare
practitioner. The author and publisher are in no way liable
for any, issue of the material.

A divine state of being, November, 2020 ©

REDISCOVERING
MY BODY

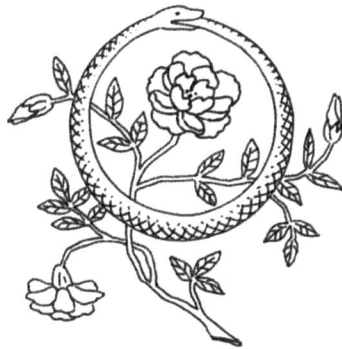

Tara Galeano

The Galeano Group

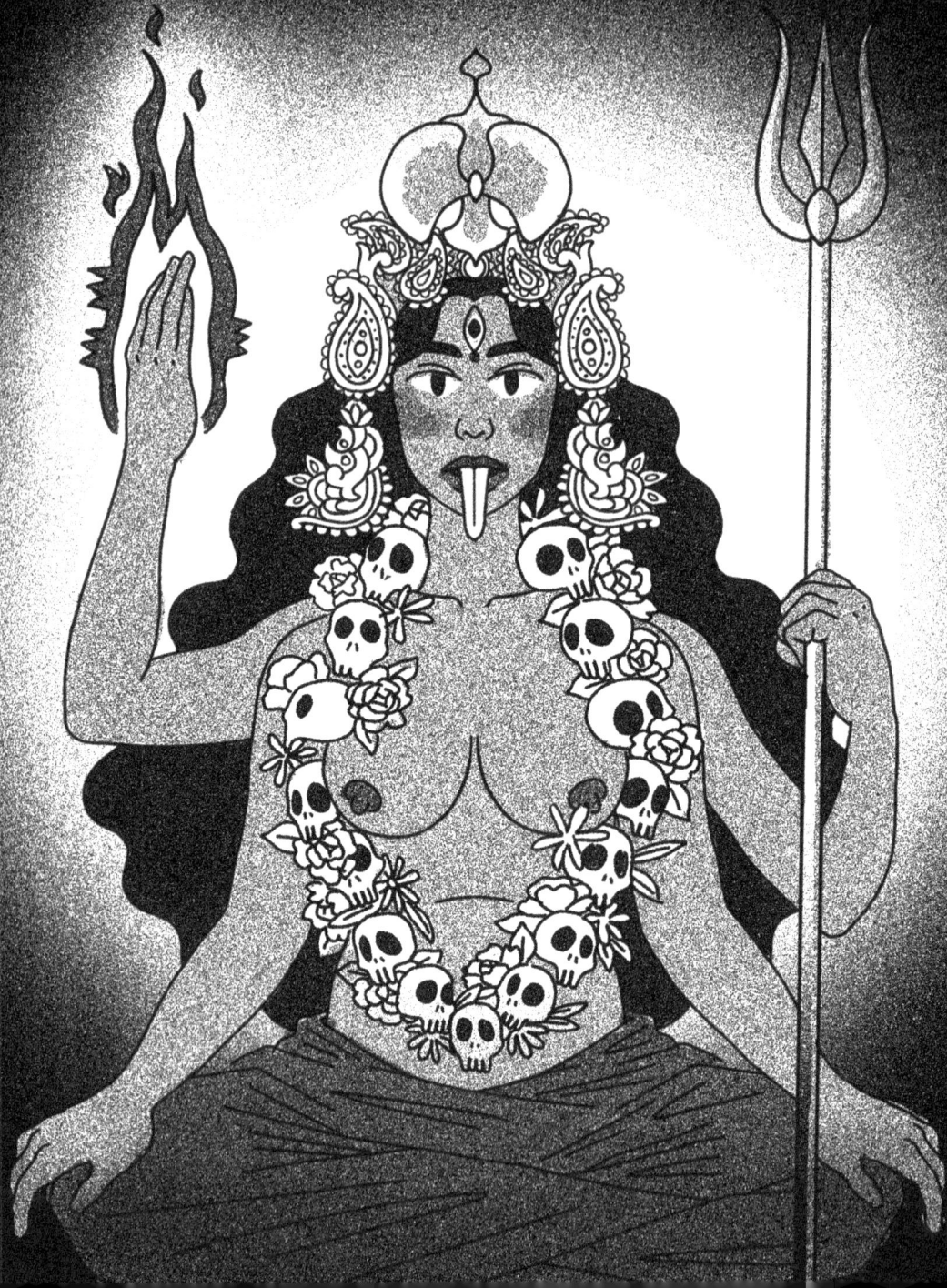

Dedication

Dedication to

The divine energy within all women that nourishes and nurtures our bodies.

This is our birthright.

It is time we know this.

Kali, goddess of fire and destruction, burning with so much love and fierceness, protect us and

help us protect.

Kali Ma, compassionately help us heal ourselves.

You are the mother of all, caring for all.

Let the healing begin here and ripple out.

Contents

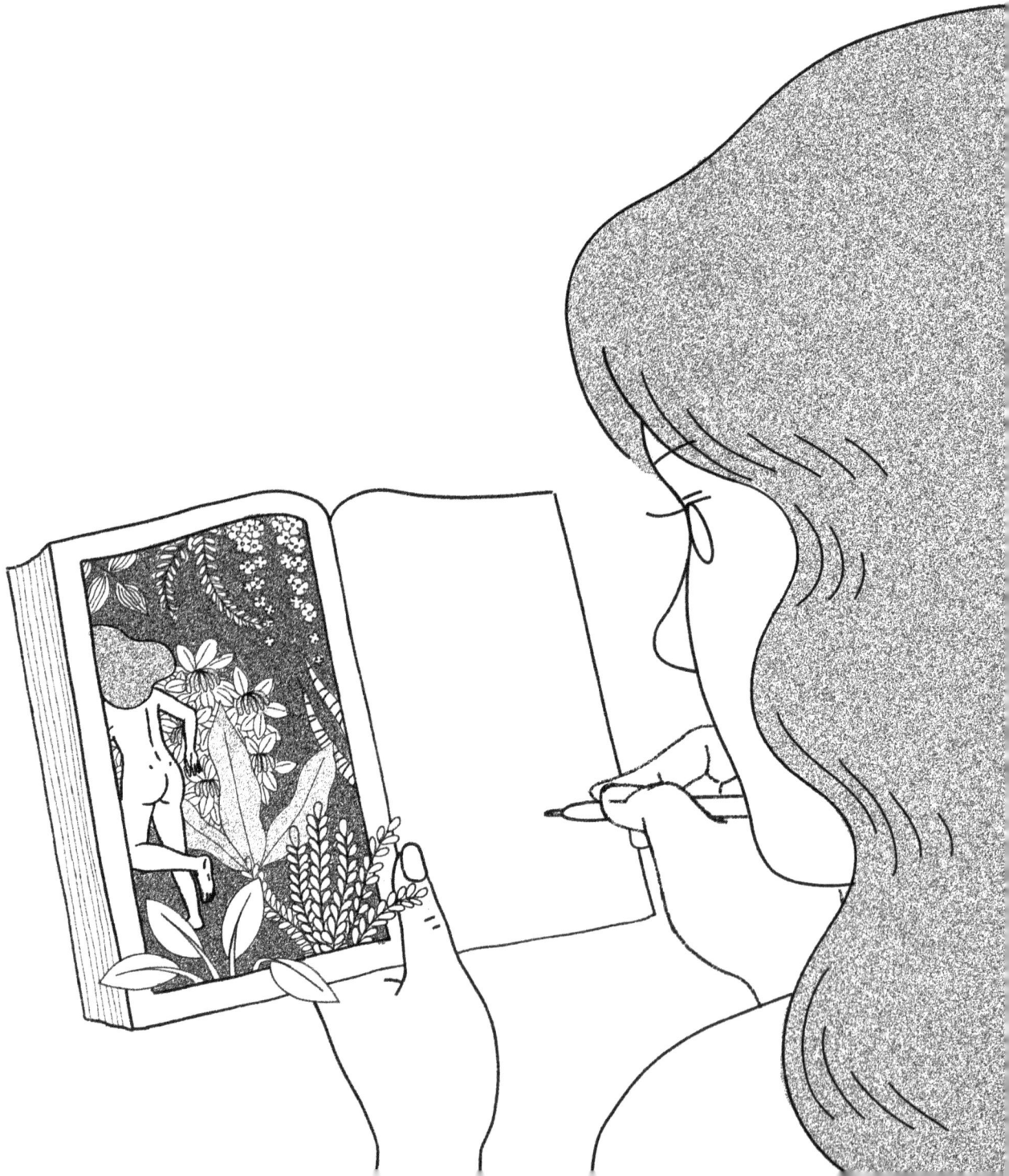

Invitation

" *Of all the art forms, poetry is the most economical. It is the one which is the most secret, which requires the least physical labor, the least material, and the one which can be done between shifts, in the hospital pantry, on the subway, and on scraps of surplus paper.*"

—Audre Lorde, *Age, Race, Class, and Sex: Women Redefining Difference*

This is a book for you. You who want to become fully enlivened sexually. Whatever your life may look like, you've decided to heal yourself—physically, mentally, emotionally, spiritually, and sexually!

Now is your time.

You can love yourself and find pleasure in the small bits and corners of your life. Sometimes that is all you have, all we have, and sometimes that's just enough.

Audre Lorde reminds you that you are the poet of your life, crafting the artistry of what it will look like from this moment forward. Embrace this idea.

Begin with Love

This is a book of love and it begins with love for yourself. You may have

scars on your body and ones in your psyche reminding you of your pain

and your experience. Your body holds so much. And now you can add

the desire to love yourself more to the top of that list of things you've

done in your lifetime. Thank Goodness.

You Are the Expert

This book is a paradigm shift. You are wise. You are whole. You are not broken.

You are declaring to the world that you want more for yourself.

This begins with you being the expert on you. Reclaim that. You are creating your solution.

This book is merely a guide. The reality is the expert is within you.

To be clear, you are the expert on you.

Suggestions on How to Use This Guidebook

This guidebook will take time to use. It may not be done in a week, although you may read it quickly. Doing the activities will take time, and it will take time to integrate them. After reading this book, it may take two weeks or a month to pick it up again and actually do an exercise. Maybe then another two weeks to try another exercise. At the same time, don't succumb to resistance and put it off because you don't want to do it. Remember—you engaged this book to become more embodied. That is your desire.

One suggestion is to read this book whole. Devour it. Know it. Consume it. Then go back to the beginning and work through the exercises sequentially, at your own pace, pausing as needed. Pauses are moments for integration. Allow that. Breathe. Allow this experience to sink deeper into the layers of your body. Feel it. Once you have acknowledged this process, proceed, or go back over it, if desired. There is no rush. Languish.

Why read it first? So your mind can wrap around the work, accept it, and ease into it. Minds need tasks. Give it this one.

Another suggestion is to just pick up the book and take off, doing each activity as it is presented. Trust the process and explore the unknown terrain, knowing that you trust yourself to pause and digest. Your approach to this book is personal. You decide.

This is a creative book. Sexuality is about imagination, playfulness, fun. This book focuses on activities that can be done alone or in community. These are not just activities but starting points for engagement, for discussion. Create language to talk about sexuality. Ignite the passion within.

Can you use this book alone? Absolutely! Can you use it with others? In a group? Go for it!

Try sharing some of these activities as it feels appropriate, maybe with a friend—a healing buddy, spiritual support, etc.

Gatherings are nourishing—women being together, creating a rhythm. In the midst of these powerful, healing women, you are supported.

Try working on each chapter over the course of a month. Maybe begin with the new moon and notice the ease of beginning events with the dark moon. Set the intention. Proceed. Give thanks. Feel.

If you choose to work with a group, try deepening with other women in the form of coming together, sharing, drawing, moving, nurturing, being nurtured, and then coming apart for a time.

Maybe try a multi-moon experience with other women, breaking down the chapters even further. Try it. You are not meant to do this life alone. Use what works best for you in the moment.

In each section, there are exercises for exploration. Try one question and answer it. Answer your own internal question as it bubbles up from within you. Recognize that if you choose to revisit this work, it may be different the next time.

Focus on personal pleasure with a journal or art diary. For journaling, you just need space. There is space. There is time. In a bounded world of time and space, go beyond.

Or set a timer, giving yourself 45 minutes for an activity and 15 minutes to debrief in your journal. An hour total.

Now you are ready to begin.

Setting the Ground, Instructions

Use this journal. Decorate it. Make it yours in your way. You are creating your guide to yourself so you will remember this path of healing. Honor it. Make it yours for future reference.

Buy some markers, watercolors, pens—ones that feel good in your hands. Test them out. What medium do you prefer? How does it feel? Create an arsenal of tools from which you can choose depending upon how you feel. Try something different.

Doodle. Decoupage. Draw. Write in this book. It is yours. It is a space in which to explore yourself.

Setting Intentions

Introduce yourself to your journal.

What do you want it to know about you?

What is important?

What can you share that you may not have with others?

This is a safe place.

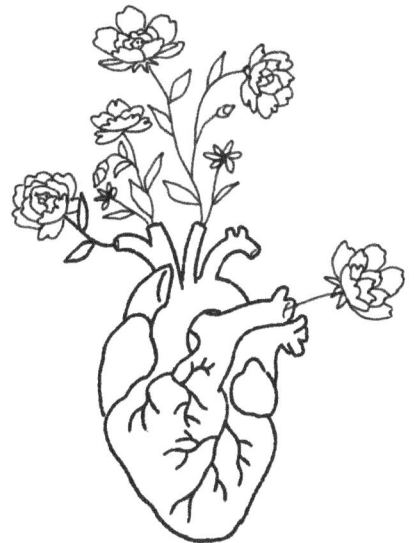

Trust YOU

This book is about trusting yourself. You decide what works for you. You know what's real for you and not someone else's agenda.

You have come here to rediscover you, now do so. Be with your tears, fears, and all.

It is a process.

This book is a gift to yourself, to share with your precious self.

This book is an invitation to help you in your healing journey. To support you in being sexual, in sexuality, and moving forward along that path, whatever that may look like today.

Why Use This Book?

Sex fortifies. You can fortify your soul through the physical replenishment of sexual connections with yourself and others.

Yet, sexual energy often lies dormant after resigning yourself to "good enough." Living in this manner, you protect yourself, wear armor, and avoid being vulnerable. As a result, you may also be bypassing your power and avoiding intimacy. Remember that intimacy begins with yourself. Begin with your physical body as the access point. Sex is physical. It is also psychological, emotional, and spiritual.

Sex deepens your sense of self. When you are ready to embrace your erotic nature, you can more completely accept different aspects of yourself. Maybe you are willing to increase your repertoire of skills to include more than the habitual ones. When you choose to embrace

your erotic nature, that commitment may take you to a place of mystery or the unknown. Go

to that place, give yourself permission.

Maybe you have experienced that you have stopped loving the preciousness of your life.

That it has fallen from your heart.

What is it like to regain your heart?

Trust.

Trust you!

It takes courage to be fearlessly, painfully in your heart. You know. You have lived to this moment and won more time here to love and live. Love and live.

Draw that invitation here.

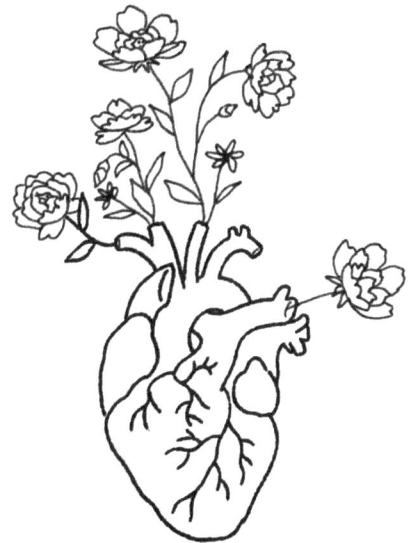

Start with your heart, yourself.

Right here.

Start here.

Draw it.

Describe it.

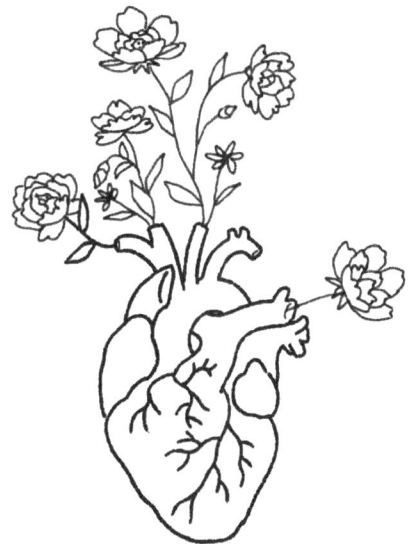

Why a Guidebook?

You are an adventurer, a brave explorer uncovering your sensuality and diving deep. Take courage to play, be creative, be imaginative in this society that demands so much of you. It is easy to play it safe. Dare to take the time for yourself, to dive into pleasure. This guidebook is for women discovering themselves in new ways. Loving themselves now, with or without a lover.

Part of this guidebook is reflective, internal work you need to do on your own. Maybe witnessed by a friend or a lover, but, ultimately, by yourself. Other parts are different. They are about techniques, trying things on, exercises, or practices that you may do more than once.

You are important, spectacular, and vital to the very fabric of the universe. How you are most fulfilled is for you to discover. Life puts you on a path of discovery. You get to choose to accept it or not. You are the most powerful agent of change in your life. Take these processes and glean what you can. You are here and resilient. Gather something good and move forward so you can continue to heal on this journey of life. REAP.

You pause all the time in your life. After a relationship. After giving birth. After a loss. These are moments in which you are deepening into just being.

How do you love yourself?

How do you love others?

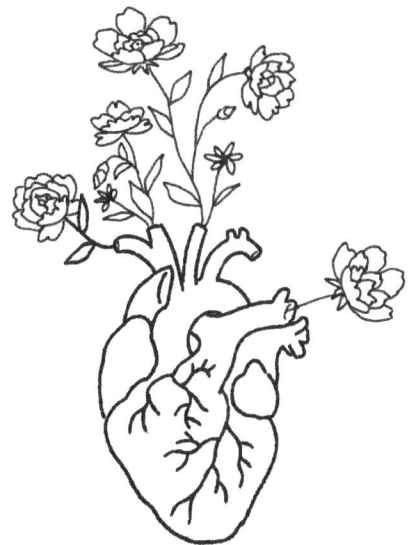

What does it mean to be sexual after a pause?

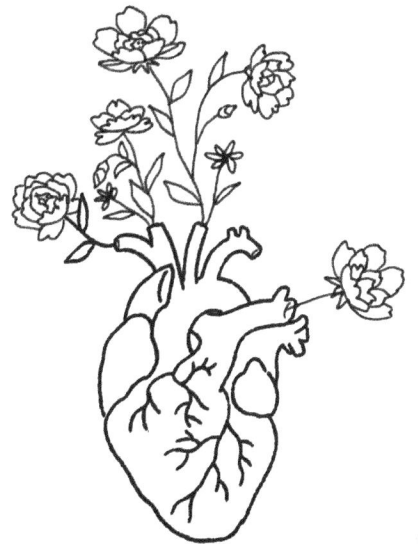

What are some of the ways that you create intimacy with yourself?

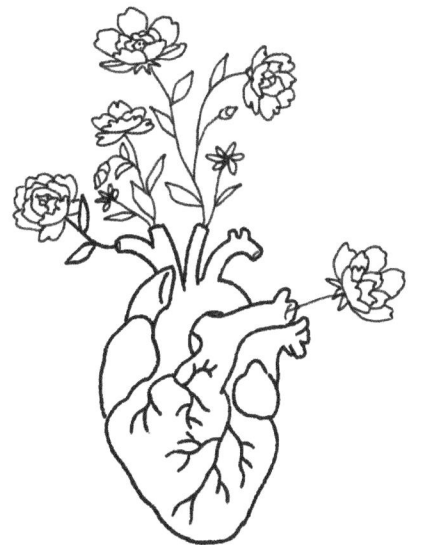

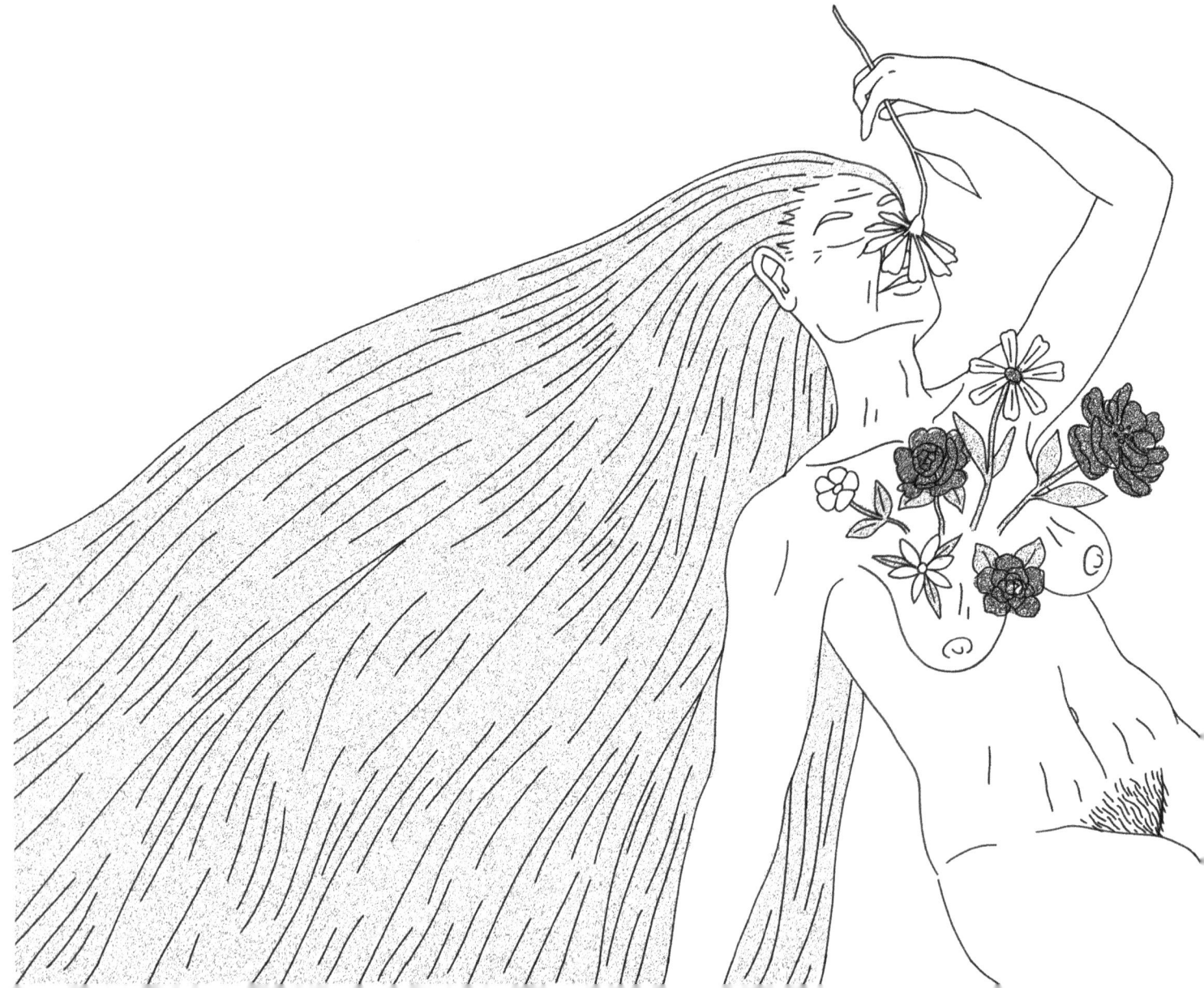

Coming Back to Your Body

"As love spontaneously wells up in us, we realize that the source of love is within us, it is always there—it is our true nature."

—Helena Meyer, Divine Path to Healing Relationships

True Intimacy

This book is about rediscovering intimacy in your life. Intimacy is often thought of as intimacy with a lover, but more importantly it is intimacy with one's self.

This is where true intimacy begins. True intimacy is the connection and ability to be with yourself in a loving, honest way.

Oftentimes, this is neglected, maybe because you didn't know it to be true. You weren't taught this.

Women are familiar with taking care of others' needs first. Throughout this book, you can begin to observe what it is like to put yourself as primary and care for yourself first. This is becoming an active agent in your life, and that leads to sexual sovereignty.

What does that look like for you?

Create that vision here.

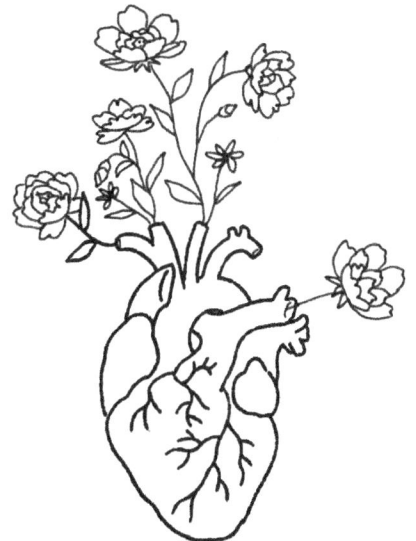

Becoming Selfish

After putting yourself on the backburner for so long, you need to learn how to be a bit more selfish. Selfish is a word that gets a bad rap. It conjures images of people who are heartless, maybe even ruthless, and do as they please without concern for others. The word for that is narcissism or possibly sociopathy: being outside of society and unable to function within it. However, being selfish has its positive and negative sides, or its sanity and neurosis, as does everything and everyone.

Try being a bit more selfish.

How does it feel?

What does it look like?

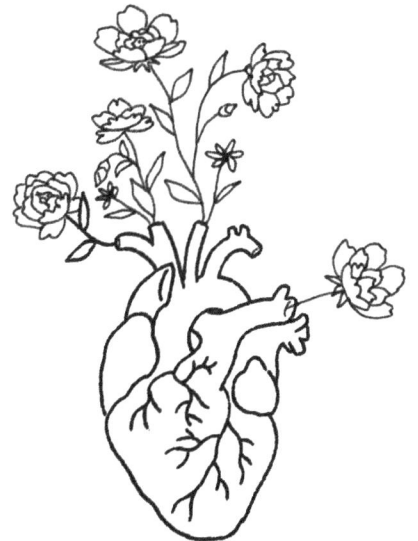

Digestion

Digestion is important. You need to "take it in." "It" being air, food, water, information, experiences. Give yourself time to digest them. Integrate them. Experience them now. Digest the experiences that you have. Allow them to be. Neither rejecting them nor denying them. Accept what was and what is.

Judgments

This is difficult work. Be brave. You'll have judgments. Be curious about your judgments. Trust yourself. Some judgments protect and others prevent you from knowing something new and exciting.

What are your judgments?

Do they need to remain at this time?

Can they be bypassed?

You decide. And realize that that too may change…

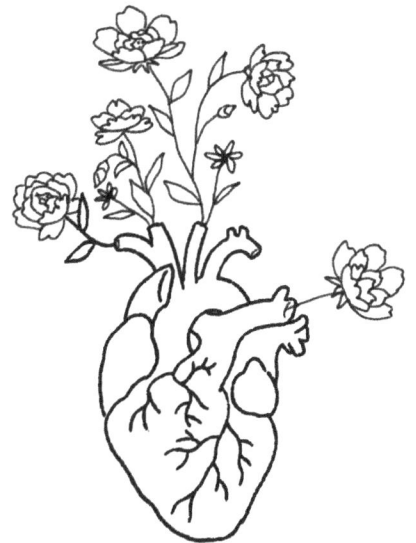

Self-noticing & Self-care

Cultivate a contemplative approach to being in the body. Notice the sensations of touch, temperature, texture, and pressure as you observe internal sensations. Begin to describe—in your own words, images, and ways—what is true for you.

Breathe deeply and exhale slowly.

Let this go.

Stand up and shake this out.

What has happened to your body as you have been reading this?

What sensations have you noticed?

Emotions?

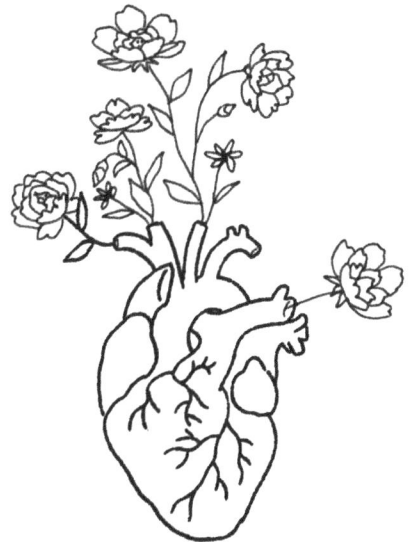

What do you need to take care of yourself?

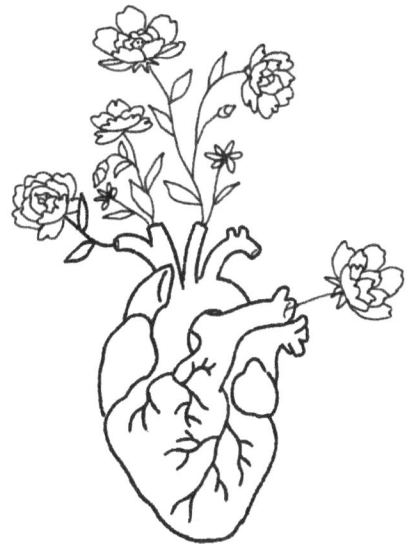

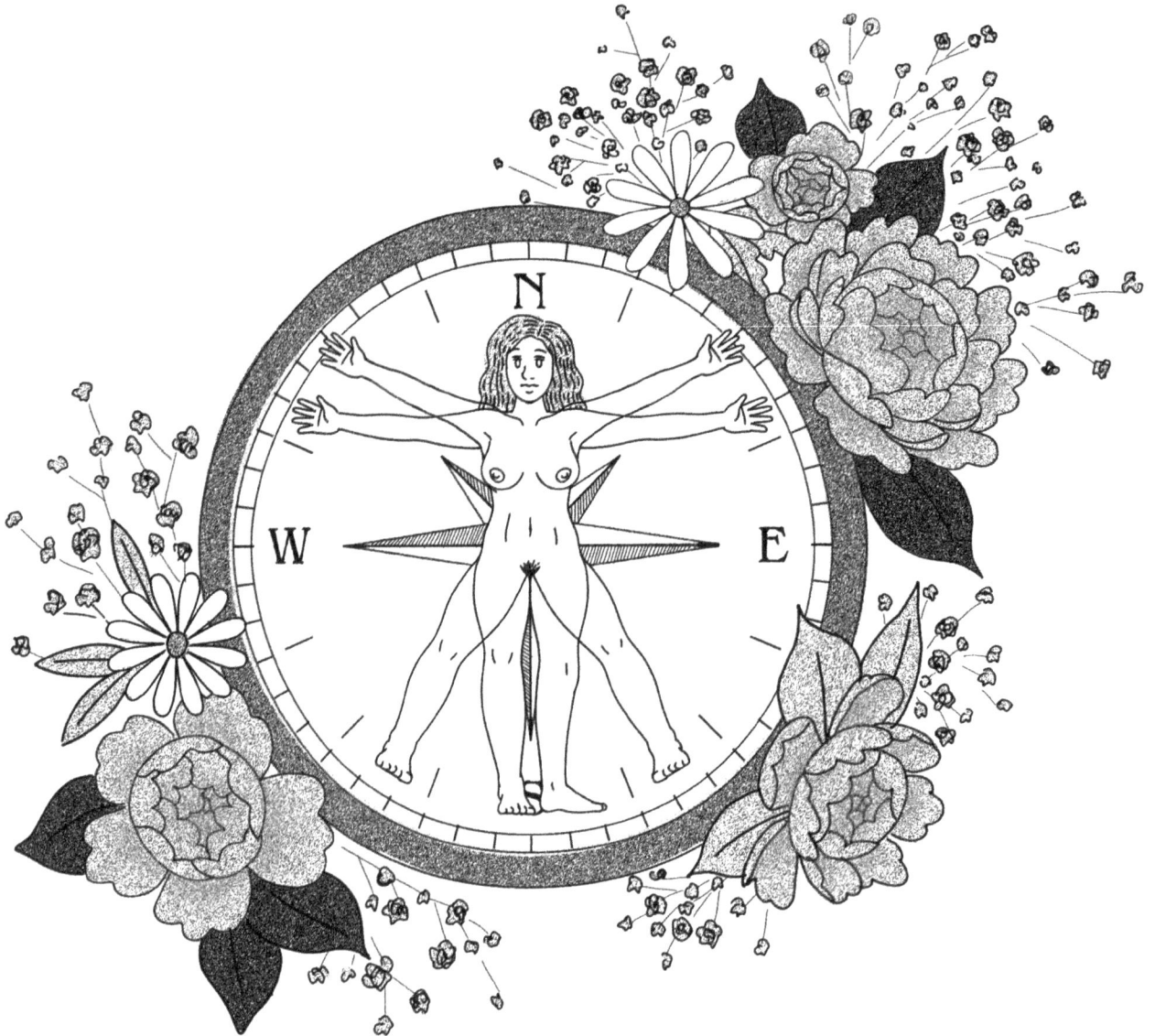

Touch, Sound, Sight

" The body never lies. "

—Martha Graham

Touch

One of the best ways to reduce anxiety is through repetitive, non-threatening, slow touch. Touch influences your well-being. Infants who are touched develop more healthily and experience fewer emotional and mental problems. Adults who are touched experience lower heart rate and blood pressure, positively impacting their immune system and promoting physical relaxation. Even petting a cat can lower a person's heart rate and blood pressure.

Being with Self

Life is a complicated journey, in which one must find their strength, touch their inner light, and love more than ever. During the course of a lifetime, you know your own fragility and mortality. You understand that time is finite. Try holding a newborn and reconnecting instantly with the preciousness of life.

When you touch yourself, do you feel that preciousness?

When did you lose that ability within yourself?

Describe a time when you noticed this.

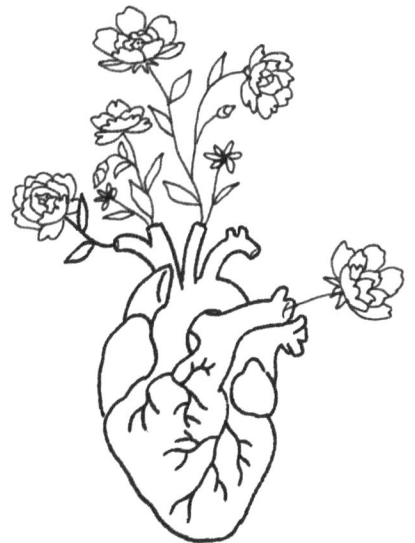

Pleasurable Touch

Touch can be the ultimate pleasure and connection. Start with yourself.

Your body needs love. Each touch may bring up a memory of a lover who touched you there. Maybe you liked the touch? Skin on skin. Contact is healing.

Touch yourself. Be safe in your body. That is something that has not always been true. You have felt fear that has made you want to run.

Self-touch begins with exploration. Every great discovery began with an adventurer. You are the explorer of your own being, of your own body. Explore the roundness. The firmness. The lumps and bumps. Feel the terrain that is yours now, not what it was so long ago or never.

You need to explore what is. You need to explore your being. Embrace it. Hold it. Love it.

This is territory to explore. Be fearless and brave. Or just love the fear, not allowing it to prevent your desire. Your desire is stronger.

Proceed with care and explore the terrain of your body. Your body now.

Your body after (fill in the blank).

How has it changed?

How has it been loved during this process?

What does it need?

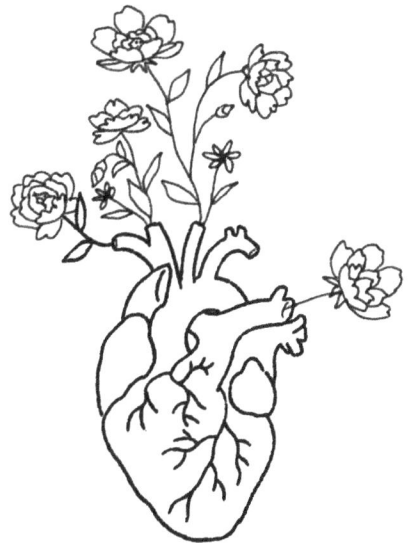

Slowly allow yourself to unfold and hear the wisdom of your words within. There is terrain to be explored that is scarred and different. Different from what you imagined it would be. Different from how you knew it before. Different. Sometimes different feels far from sexy.

Touch yourself. Understand the art of self-pleasure. Feel into the body. Touch your body. Check in. Suspend judgment. Be curious if you notice it arising. What is that about? There is no need to react. If it persists, how do you honor it?

How do you say, "I trust myself"? Say "I trust myself" out loud. Say "This doesn't feel right. I feel it in my gut." Both of these statements suspend judgment. Trust yourself as you engage your curiosity. Be true to yourself. Be your new self—whatever that may look like. Allow it to emerge. Be gentle with your body.

Touch is healing. Touch yourself.

You are your own first healer. You can heal through pleasure, through self-love. Gently touch yourself all over. Feel your fingertips on your toes. Use some oil. Make it soothing. Maybe this is your first time touching yourself. Just touch and explore. Try 20 minutes of skin stimulation, without genital contact, by yourself.

Now.

Where are your erogenous zones?

How many do you have?

Stop and count them.

Draw a picture of them here.

Try drawing what they look like as they are gently stroked.

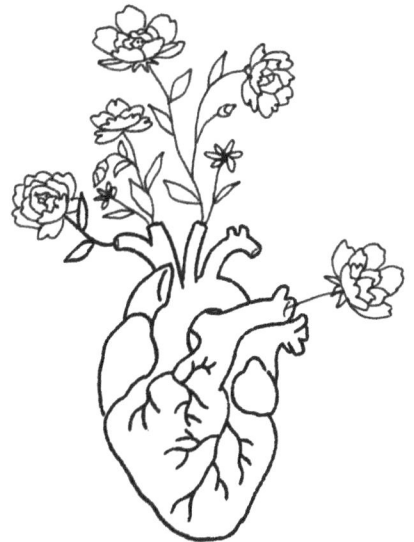

Breath

Another way to touch yourself internally is through deep, slow, rhythmic breathing. Inhale through the nose, slowly exhale through the mouth, preferably making a sound. Try that now. Come back to the body. Notice how it has been rejected. Explore it. Inhale. Exhale. Exhale longer. Know your breath. Come back to your body. Feel your breath.

Remember to be mindful. Love your body first. Know that that is most important. Rest, relax, eat healthy nutritious meals. Lie in the sun, exercise—walk, bike, swim, lift weights, do yoga. Do what you love. Move your body, dance, make love. Sleep. Engage in restorative activities. Ayurveda states that sex is one of the three pillars of life. The others are food and sleep. Restore yourself by honoring these three pillars.

Sound

Consider the sound that touches your ears. It is important. Soothing, prosodic tones heal your being. Infants respond to soft, soothing voices. Loud, blaring, metal guitars do not put a child to sleep. They are not soothing. They create disturbances in the child's nervous system.

What soothes your nervous system?

What is prosodic to your soul?

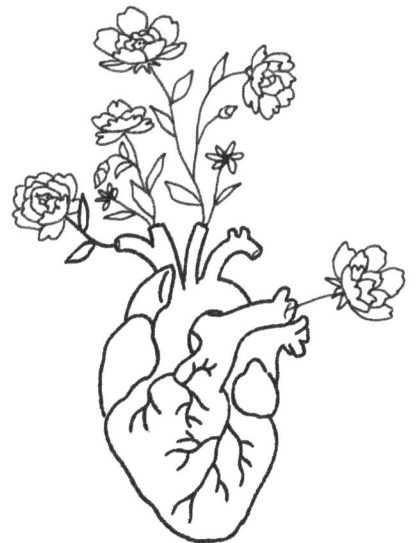

Music may help you understand how to get into that space of healing, of knowing, of pleasure.

What are your creature comforts?

Music and movement? Stillness?

What emerges from that still place within?

Listen.

What do you hear?

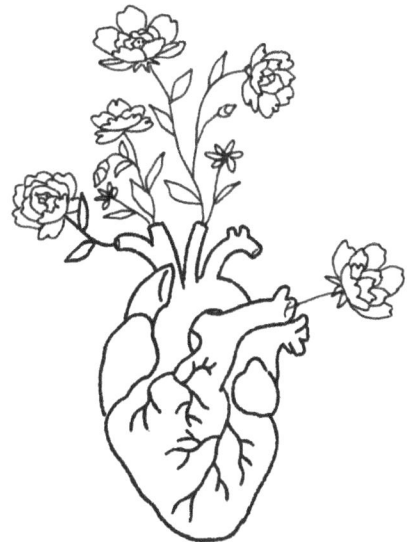

Sight

What you think you're supposed to look like and what you actually look like is a very fertile place for self-doubt and shame to grow, often impeding intimacy. As difficult as it is to open up to someone, it's even harder when you feel desperate to hide, particularly in the bedroom. Shame and anxiety about one's body leads to the avoidance of physical closeness and reduces sexual satisfaction. Poor body image equates with low self-esteem and low confidence, which means you don't feel sexy. If you don't like the way you look, you aren't going to have megawatt sex.

You live in this body, every day. You watch it change, grow older. Perceptions differ with time. Sex is about being embodied.

"Women with poor body image don't initiate sex as often, and they're more self-conscious,"

Ann Kearney-Cooke, PhD, director of the Cincinnati Psychotherapy Institute.

If you're preoccupied with your body, you obviously won't be focusing on your desires or anyone else's, or be present in the moment, for that matter.

How does body image facilitate sex?

How does it inhibit it?

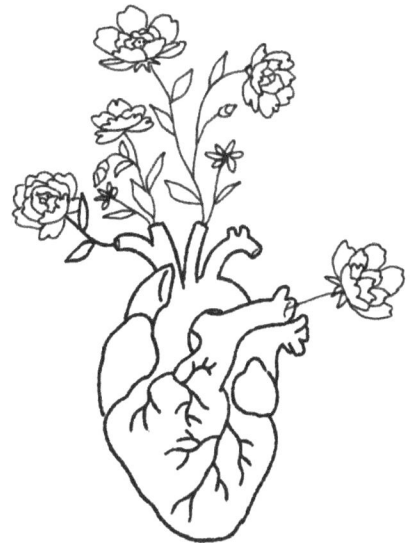

Does this feel true for you?

How can you receive pleasure, or give pleasure to yourself, if you don't like the way you look?

If what you see turns you off?

How does that impact how you feel?

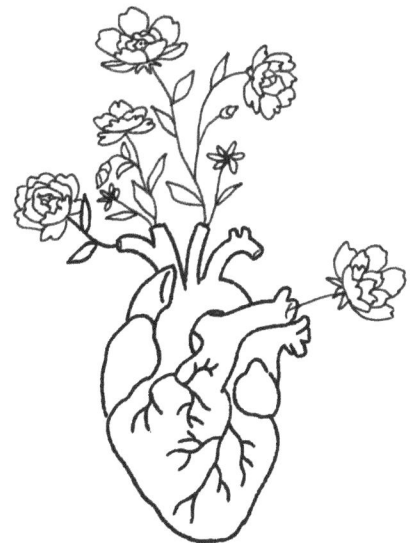

Body Map

You'll need help with this. Have someone you trust outline your body with clothes on. Ask them to draw a line around the outside of your body, over your head, around your fingers, in between your legs. Uncomfortable or exciting? Either way, have them outline your body so you can see as much of you as possible. See yourself within the lines.

Ask your friend to leave you alone as you work on yourself. Create a legend to your map. Write the key to yourself. Fill in the space. For example, use flowers for pleasure, red for pain. Mark erogenous zones with a bull's eye. Or use a colored marker to block off areas of your body that are off limits. Use a different marker for areas where you experience pleasure. Be as creative as you like. Be the artist you are.

Fill in the space and notice where there is still space. Let it be. Focus on how you are in this moment. Not on how you or your body was or how you'd like it to be, but on how it is. Take time. Be with yourself.

Try again. Redraw the outline. Remember to love yourself.

Date your outlines. Let them go.

What has changed? It is not you, but an image.

Hug yourself.

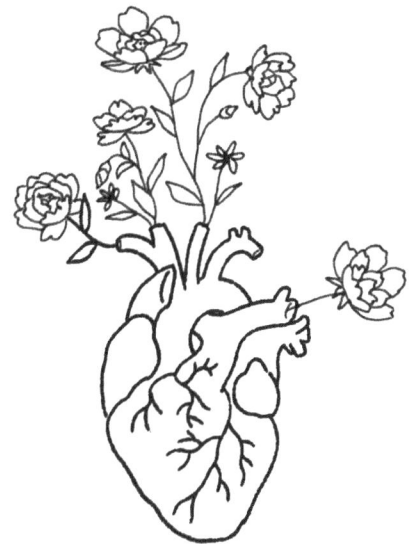

When you are ready, share the outline with another—maybe the person who outlined you, maybe not. You are brave. You are here. You are doing this. It can be scary. That's okay. You are intact. Friends are supportive and love you.

Show a lover. That can be scarier. Let them know what feels good and what doesn't feel good. You are vulnerable. They want to know. They want to be able to touch you in a way that pleases you. That is best. To be touched. Love it.

To truly communicate is risky. Take risks. This may be difficult. Feel vulnerable. Feel sadness. Feel what you feel. Tears are okay. Let them go. Let them wash over your face—cleanse, purify. Make mistakes. Are you understood? Try again. That is all you can do.

You shared your outline. Success.

Stand in front of a full-length mirror. Start fully clothed. Take a moment. Drink yourself in. Look. Examine. See what you look like in all your clothes. See what others may see. Get a glimpse. Process it. Digest it. Let it be.

Try this again. Take your time. Stay longer. Time yourself if needed. Five minutes, now ten minutes.

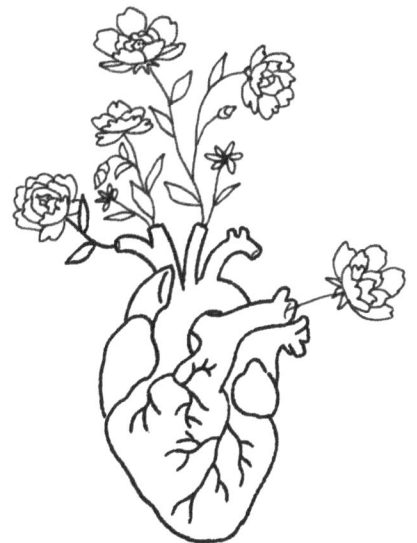

Mirror Gazing Without Clothes

Unfold into the next part. Try taking your clothes off. Get naked. Examine your nakedness. Turn around. Use a full-length mirror. View you. Revel in you.

Begin small, but begin. How about your nose? This side. That. Inside. Out. The area around your nose. Your cheeks. Skin. The blackheads. The pores. Notice. Microscopic. Pull away. See your face. Face your face. Drink it in. Can you dare love it? What do you love? What do you see? Must you blink? Can you stare? For how long? When does the love leave your eyes? Does it ever get there? Curious. Curiosity. Where is that? Tell me. Take a break. Write it down. Dance. Express.

Scream.

Resume. What more can you take in? What's easy? Elbows? Feet? Ears? What do you like? What do you avoid? What brings tears? Breathe. Be. Know love. Be. Rest when you need. Love yourself as you love yourself. Touch yourself softly. Be gentle with yourself. Stroke gently down and away from your heart. Speaking love or just feeling. Noticing. That's it.

Hold a hand-held mirror over yourself. Get comfortable. Change positions. Allow it to be. Ease into it. Change positions again. Adjust. Get comfortable. Hold the mirror so you can see your vulva, your external genitalia.

Look at yourself.

How was that?

Write about it.

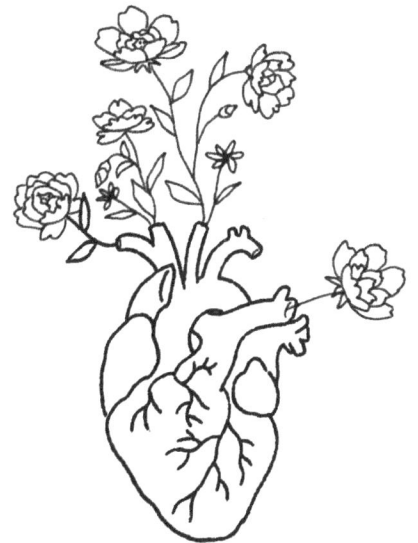

Develop the witness, the observer within. Notice what arises in your body.

The sensations. Notice the pleasure. What co-exists?

How do you limit pain and/or pleasure?

How do you experience them both?

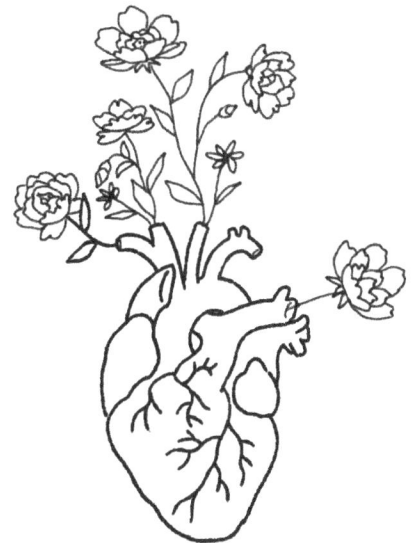

What will it be like next time?

Next time you allow yourself.

Is there discomfort and pain being in your body?

Tightness or swelling?

How will you work with the truth?

Your truth?

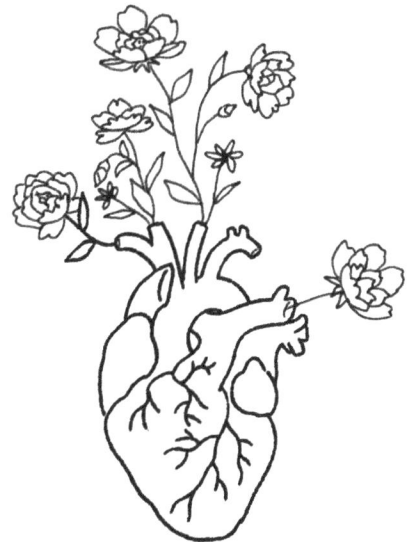

First Sex

What was it like the first time? What did it mean the first time?

What does it mean now? What constitutes a first time? What did you imagine?

Was it pain tinged with pleasure or pleasure tinged with pain?

Share with yourself what it was. What it will be.

Write it down. Capture it. Remind yourself.

Remember. Allow yourself to revisit this exercise.

It was real. It is real.

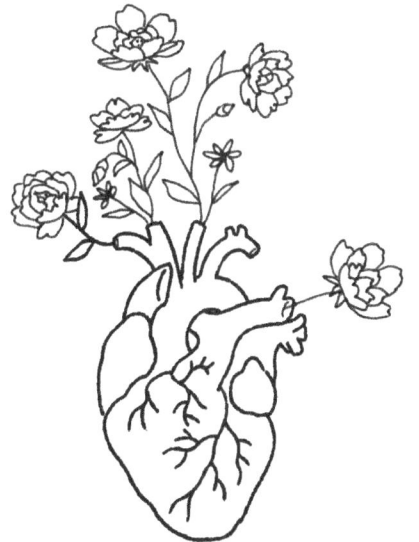

Focus on the physical sensations. Allow them to be. Untethered in your mind. Then localized again in your body. It's okay. Breathe. Feel the pain. Feel the pleasure. Stop if it becomes too much. But feel it. Practice not avoiding or indulging. Touch into it. Feel it. Let it go. It is there. It needs attention. Both may need attention—pleasure and pain. One will subside. The other will dominate. Let that be okay. Stop if it overwhelms you. You are in charge of this experience.

Experience it with all your body, your skin, your movement. Is there a sound to make? Okay.

Let it be. Now try a movement with the sound. What does that feel like? You are okay. Just

experience. Allow yourself the pleasure and the pain. Pain is part of life. Physical pain.

Emotional pain. Psychological pain. It persists, aiding trauma. Know that you can heal, sex is

pleasure.

Sex is healing. Have an orgasm a day. How does that help with pain management? Feel.

I want to tell you about the pleasures of just receiving and the clitoral stimulation that can bring you ecstasy. This is important because women have trouble receiving. This is a practice. Try it alone. Try it with your partner. Notice. Observe. Be one with that pleasure. Feel the reverberations throughout your body. Good. Just allow it to be. It is important. The powerful healing orgasm. You can read more about different types of orgasms or clitorises and vulvas later. The names are not important, but the feelings are. The names are only important as you claim your words, create your language.

Keep a self-pleasure journal. Wow! Write an entry for each day. Engage yourself each day so that you know pleasure. Capture it via text, audio file, or in a traditional journal.

Your Sex Story

Sex is fun. Being sexual can be wet, wild, and exciting. Try it on. Dive into your body. Try what

you like. Try something new. Before you begin, consider:

What is sex? What is pleasure?

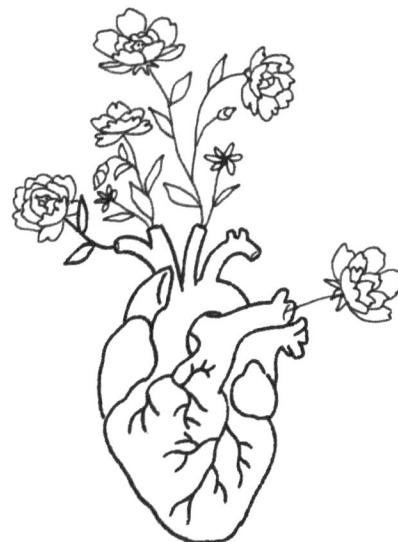

What makes sex meaningful? What makes it good?

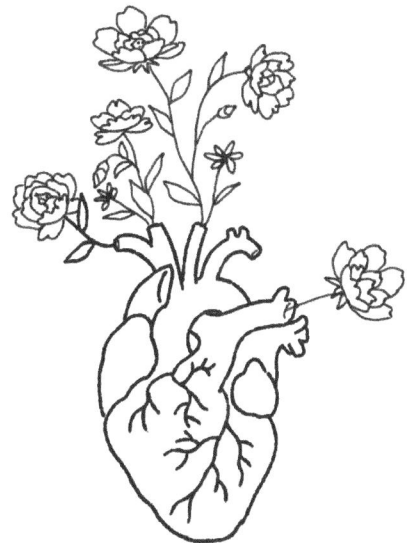

What is it like today?

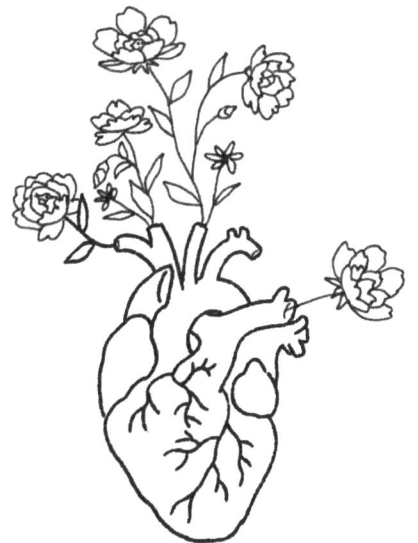

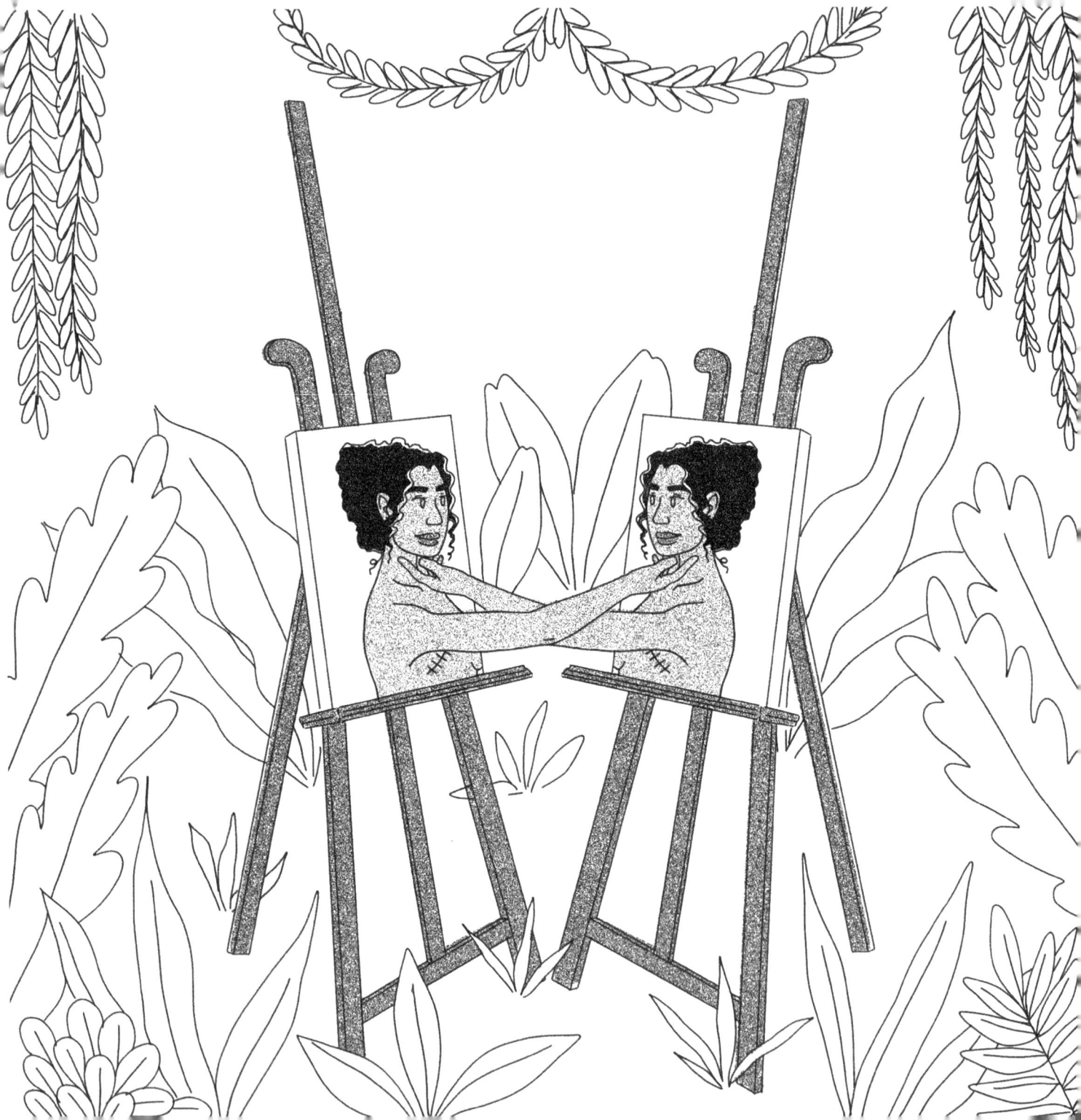

Trusting Yourself

" I paint self-portraits because I am so often alone, because I am the person I

know best. "

—Frida Kahlo

Sometimes you feel that you have no control. When life hits, you may feel lost. "How has this happened?" "Why?" You feel incredulous. "What to do?" "Tell me the way," you ask. It often appears as if the answer is not within. You are guided by others. Professionals who aid. Peers who support. That may feel like the best route. They know something that maybe you don't.

STOP HERE FOR A MOMENT.

Take three deep breaths. Stop listening to everyone else. Listen to yourself now.

What about your own internal connection?

How do you perceive truth in your body?

What do you feel in your body?

What is it telling you?

Is there a disconnect?

Notice the sensations.

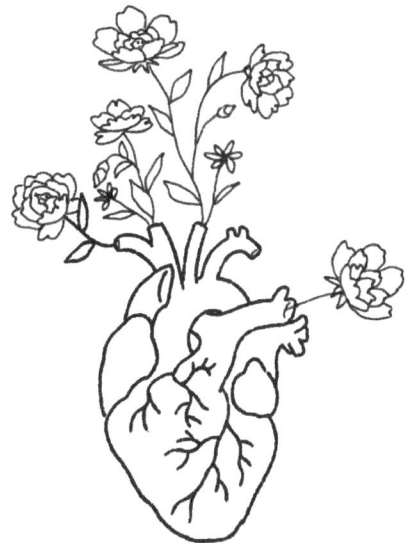

Changes in Your Body

As a woman, your body is constantly changing, as are your perceptions of it. Changes in your body happen as you age, are pregnant, go through menopause, etc. Add what you like to the list. Framing these experiences as change, well, isn't that sugar-coating or minimizing your experience? Allow yourself to know this process. Give yourself permission to feel—sad, depressed, angry, powerful, elated—as you evolve with experience.

Feeling the Experiences of Life

Let yourself feel the fullness of you. Whatever that looks like. When change happens, you are presented with opportunities that are both known and unknown. That can bring up fear. How will you proceed? What will you do?

What did you notice in your body as you read this?

Maybe nothing. Maybe something to dismiss.

But when you feel it, what is it?

Admit this to yourself.

Create this alliance within.

It is safe here.

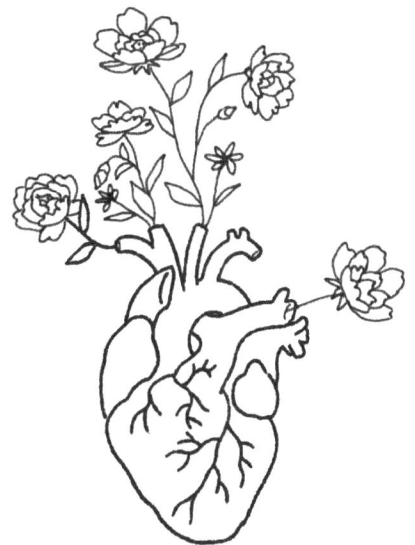

Autonomic Nervous System

The autonomic nervous system (ANS) runs throughout your body, through your nerve endings. It is also called the involuntary nervous system. The ANS provides nerves to your internal organs, i.e. heart, diaphragm, intestines, stomach, and genitals. You don't have much control over the responses of any of these organs. For example, food in the stomach triggers a series of reflexes involved in digestion. The same is true of stimulation of the vagina, which causes lubrication.

The autonomic nervous system has two divisions—the sympathetic nervous system (SNS) and the parasympathetic nervous system (PNS).

The SNS is responsible for initiating the stress response, which functions to expend energy rapidly, think fight or flight. In this stress response, your eyes dilate, your heart pounds, and the blood rushes away from the center of your body to your limbs so you can run or fight.

The PNS has the opposite function—to conserve energy. It is in charge of the relaxation response. PNS controls the early stages of arousal. It is responsible for the freeze in the fight, flight, or freeze response.

Anxiety occurs when something real or perceived threatens your life. You cannot be both anxious and relaxed at the same time.

Restoration of the nervous system begins simply. Curl up on your side and rest with your arm in the crook of your neck. Lie with your knees tucked in a fetal position. Rest here. Try this now.

Knowing Your Gut

Learn to consider this impulse in your gut. That is part of loving yourself. Learning slowly

what it means to care for your being. We make mistakes. Mistakes sometimes make a pattern.

Notice. Catalog your gathered and learned skills. Recognize your mastery over behaviors that

no longer serve or are no longer required. Life has changed. You have evolved beyond the

pattern. You are ready to make new decisions, new choices. Sometimes this is not even on

a conscious level, but you feel in your gut that you need to do something different, create

something different. The old way no longer serves you. Grow. Change. Make a different choice

informed by your gut. You decide. Try something new.

Come back to your gut. Notice what happens in your body. The nervous system can get overloaded—usually unintentionally, sometimes intentionally. Maybe there is disassociation, numbness, blockage.

It is easier to bypass being in the body. This is real. It happens all the time. Forgetting the body, you become a head (bodiless being) for a time. Come back to the body.

The pain of trauma also deeply delves into communities. Its reverberations ripple through the heart and body of towns, cities, and countries. When trauma can no longer be ignored, it must be addressed. It is pervasive.

Grounding Next to a Tree

Lie down next to a tree. Feel the ground beneath you. Observe the clouds. You are supported. You are loved. The earth is there to support you. Hold you. Heal you. Let any tension in your body melt down into the earth. The feelings release. Any tension. Any tightness. Let it go. Let it be. Release. Be with the earth. Feel. Love that release. Your body image comes into your mind. Let that go. You think you know your body. You think you know. You think. No body, just a head. Head, no body. Bodiless head floating in your perception. Being self. Being with a tree. Being a tree. Let It Go. Let It Go. Love. Relief. Love yourself. Love yourself. What do you experience? What can you share?

Body Scan

Sit on your chair with your feet flat on the floor. Your arms and legs uncrossed, sitting up straight with your hands in your lap. Be comfortable. Put a pillow behind your back. Relax and notice. Read these instructions once then try it.

Bring your attention to the top of your head. Slowly bring your attention down your body, from the top of your head to your face, your neck, your chest, etc. Slowly bring your awareness to any tension in your body and just notice. There is no need to change anything, just note what you feel and continue to bring your awareness down to your toes.

Imagine your body. Close your eyes. Scan your body by feeling your body internally. Start at the top. Feel any sensations. Notice any tension. Let it melt away. You are aware. You are letting go. Continue to move down your body. Feel the tension melting, leaving your body. Going into the earth. Continue to notice. Continue.

Use a body scan every time you begin your work with this guidebook. Become familiar with the process. Be in your body. Notice. Be aware. Love. Good. Down to your toes. Breathe. Inhale. Exhale. Let the exhalation guide the tension out of your body. You are okay. Good.

Record your voice guiding you through this process. Make it your own.

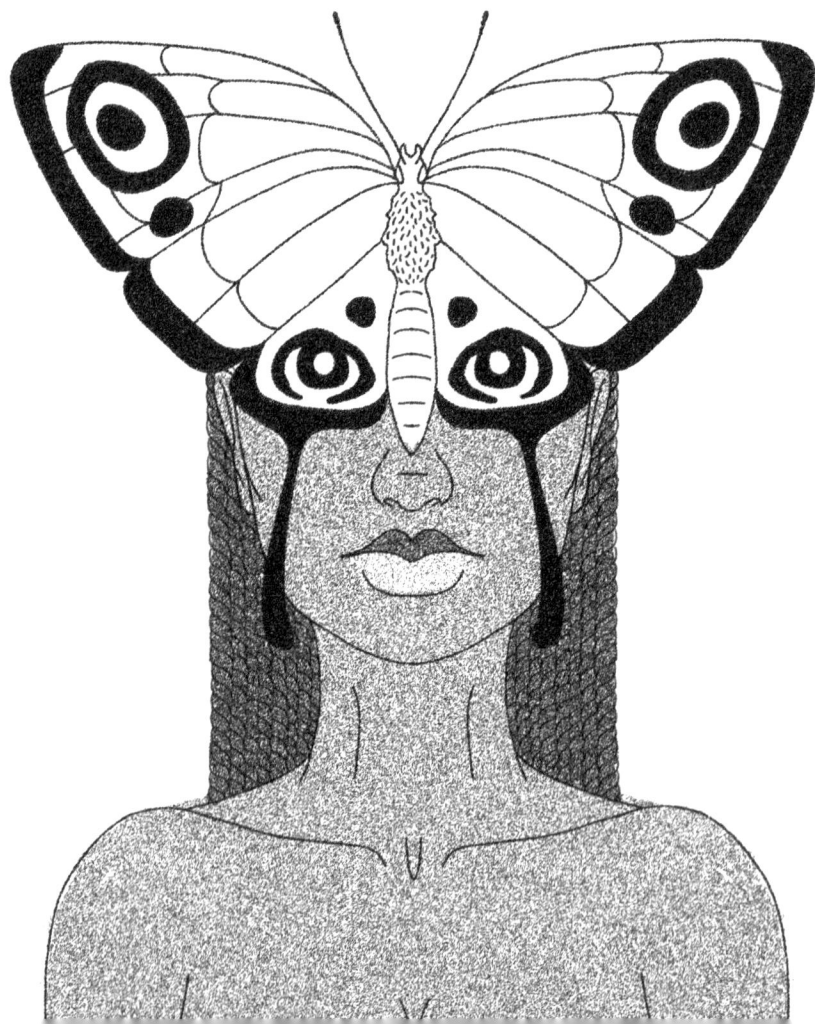

Knowing Your Emotions

" We delight in the beauty of the butterfly, but rarely admit the changes it

has gone through to achieve that beauty. "

—*Maya Angelou*

Emotions and Feelings

Emotions are physical, intense, and shorter in duration than feelings. They are messengers that create sensations to help us understand how we feel. Feelings may be more cerebral in nature. Opening up the heart allows energy to flow so you can embrace life. Feeling is important. It opens your heart.

Imagine a time when you were sad. Describe the experience.

What were the physical sensations?

How long did that experience last?

Which does it feel more like—a feeling or an emotion?

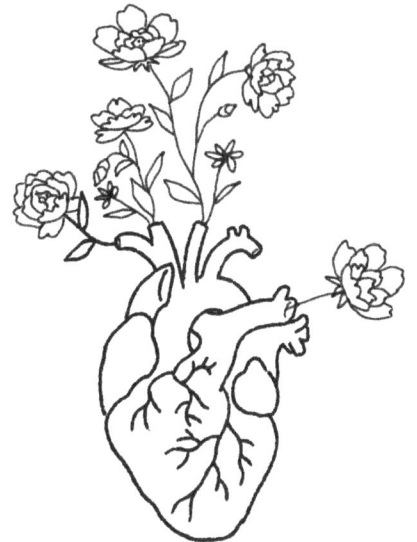

Grief

Rediscovering intimacy begins when you acknowledge that you have experienced a loss—due to divorce, empty nest, chronic illness, relocation, etc. Loss is real. With loss, you grieve. You let go. There may also be struggle with grief. Denial. You can't believe what has happened. You feel you have less time. Less time to give, less time to share, less time for yourself, and no time for one more thing.

There may be layers of grief, soft like lace obscuring what is underneath, or thick and opaque. Notice. Tears roll down your face. Let the tears roll for whatever sadness or sorrow they hold. Any shame or fear they contain, just let it go. Tears release. Let them go. No need to be contained. They are rinsing your face clean. Releasing. Tears are cleansing, then gone. Allow them. Observe them. Tears come or not. And that's okay too.

Grieving is a process. How do you give yourself time to grieve? How do you give yourself permission to just be with grief? Especially when there are so many demands on you. Sometimes it is difficult or confusing to just be. If you allow yourself to just be, you may never get out of bed, let alone have pleasure in your body.

Grieving is not a linear experience and there may be repetition in the sequence. Yes, this again. You have time. Each breath is another moment you are alive, and now is the time. Time to heal. Time to grieve. Time to rediscover.

Grief can be an obstruction, but it doesn't have to be. It can be effectively worked with, and needs to be to move on. Grief creates a deep hole in your heart where you may want to bury a part of yourself—in this case, maybe a relic of yourself that was "happier," "more whole," or just "more sexual." You can get stuck in the comparison.

Grief also creates a softness, a vulnerability, where you can connect with others. It is only through your vulnerability that you truly connect with another intimately. Be gentle and tread wisely. Grief is an immense opportunity, but very painful.

Grief changes you neurally. That is profound. Grief dampens your neurotransmitters and darkens your view of the world, of your life. It is a pervasive experience that changes your perception of what can be. Grief comes; it subsides and it comes again. Over time, it lessens. Acknowledge and work with the grief of your loss—the full impact of grief. You have a life. You have a voice. You have a body. You have your loves. You are alive. Enough. Yet there is grief. Let this be.

Shame

Shame often blends into the development of our sexual selves. Sometimes it begins as the shame of being sexual, of coming of age, then it progresses from there. Positive role models who are comfortable and ordinary with their sexuality are few and far between. Be brave and be curious about your shame as it arises. Trust yourself. Observe. Try not to react; notice.

You may be struggling with shame—both the shame of being and the shame of being sexual. Brene Brown says, "Shame is the intensely painful feeling that you are unworthy of love and belonging."

Shame is often accompanied by judgments—yours or another's judgments that have been internalized. Sometimes they constrict you and prevent you from trying something new.

Judgments can also be present to protect.

What are your judgments? Do they need to stay in place now?

Can you put them aside? How would that work?

Where do you feel that in your body?

Notice it. Bring attention there.

Love it. Honor it.

This is the process—again and again.

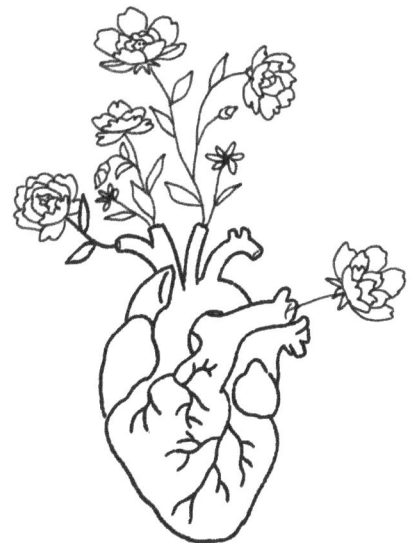

Self-aggression

Once shame has been recognized, often there is mobilization to eradicate it. "I don't want to feel that." Shame is traded for self-aggression. Aggression is painful. Try being with the process. What dissolves? There is no need to rush forward because you desire progress and change and heal. That is aggression. Approach each day, each moment, with resolve. You're moving forward, in the present, moment by moment. This is how to heal. First, you must feel Aggression towards pain, even to make it go away, is just more self-aggression. Observe it. Be with it. Breathe into it. It will pass. Pain is impermanent; most feelings are. Pain is temporary, even the chronic variety. There are moments when your pain subsides. Your awareness shifts to something else. Take it moment by moment.

Observe the pain. Where is it located?

Where does it exist?

The pain has an ending point,

a location in your body.

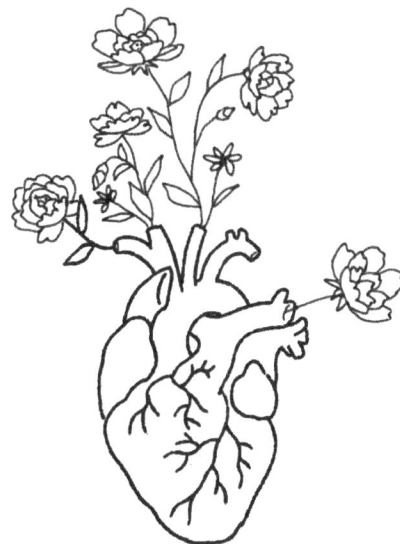

How is that? Breathe into that. Feel it.

Pain in my (name your body part)

is (fill in the blank).

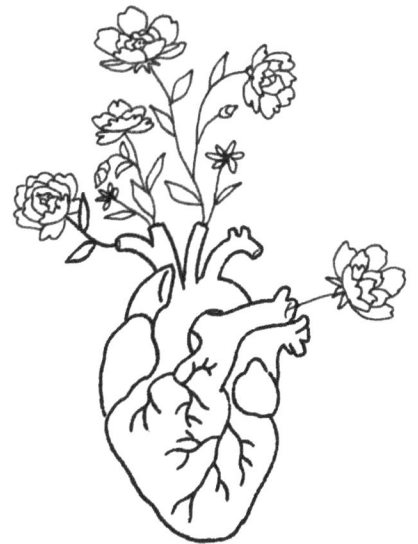

Feel its temperature. Is it cold? Hot? Feel its texture. Is it smooth? Rough? Bumpy? Sharp? Does it radiate? How may your curiosity grow? Observe it. You are creating more awareness and are able to observe more sensations. That is key. Congratulations.

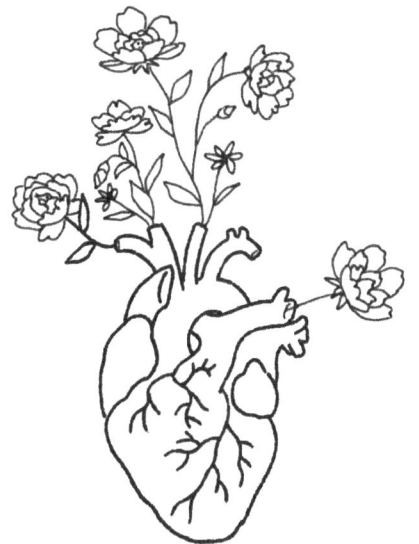

Transforming Aggression Through Awareness

Notice the aggression. Meditation, a contemplative practice, is helpful for observation. Awareness increases with meditation. Mindfulness is another form of contemplative practice. Both help heal and improve awareness of the physical body—sex, sexuality, sensuality. You can change. You are changing. A mentor said that therapy is about creating greater options because your view has expanded. There is more breadth.

Awareness helps.

Trade in your aggression for awareness. Through awareness, you can make different choices. Awareness of the body begins with noticing the sensations. Notice the breath. Notice how you feel in your body. You are blessed to have a body and awareness. Awareness is perception.

Perception may be judged as good or bad. Feel the pain in your body. Feel the blockages. Pain that keeps you up at night, that impedes your imagination, blocking everything—pleasure, sex, being sexual. As much as you can be with the pain, be with it. Don't push it away. Don't avoid it. Acknowledge it. Don't judge it. It just is. Good.

A Word About Anxiety

The amygdala, the part of the brain that controls fear and anxiety, needs to be put to rest before you can respond sexually. Your partners' bad breath, slobber, and/or clumsy moves can reactivate the amygdala, short-circuiting your sexual interest. Bad past experiences can start to occupy your brain, activating the amygdala—shame, awkwardness, lack of safety, lack of confidence, etc. Truly, your mind is the most important sex organ.

"Basically, you need to be in a good mood before sex."

—Dr. Brizendine, author of The Female Brain.

Anger at one's partner is one of the most common reasons for sexual problems. However, most women can't be angry at their partner and want to have sex with them at the same time.

There is a window of opportunity! This begins twenty-four hours before sexual activity.

Anxiety is the biggest cause of sexual problems. Reducing anxiety is crucial for sexual healing to occur. Noted.

Sex is and can be out of control. Oftentimes you have a sense of wanting to control. Your body is alive and does not follow dictates that you may have in your mind about what is appropriate.

Can you be with a loss of control?

How does it feel when you are out of control?

How are you with that?

Is there anxiety?

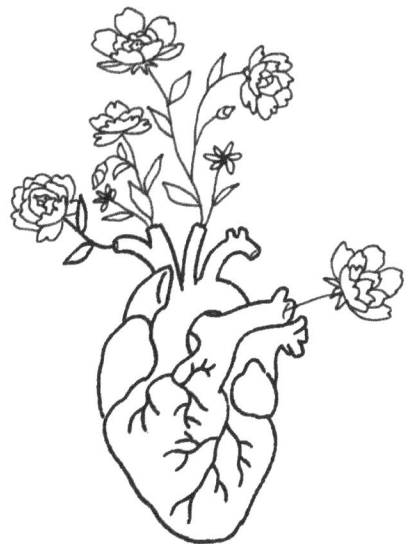

Anger & Rage

Anger is caused by a violation of a boundary or agreement. It is regulated by your parasympathetic nervous system. You get angry. An agreement has been broken. You speak up.

Rage is a self-protective mechanism that is regulated by your sympathetic nervous system. Rage is driven by a survival impulse from your limbic brain.

Rage is out of control because you feel the real or perceived threat that you need to protect yourself from at whatever cost. Rage is beyond anger. To be stuck in rage can cause heaviness. Observe this.

Rage may be explosive. You are shaking. This is the culmination of all the threats that you have endured. There is rage. THERE IS RAGE! Rage is scary. Rage can't be controlled. It is volatile.

It exists and you shudder.

 How can this be good? You wish it was something else. You desire to be something you are currently not. You push away the rage. Shut it down. Self-aggression or self-preservation. Which is it?

 Rage is difficult to navigate. "I am afraid to be with my body because of all the rage it holds. I was violated. I feel rage." How to be with that?

Where is that rage in your body?

What does it look like?

What does it feel like?

Is it hot or cool?

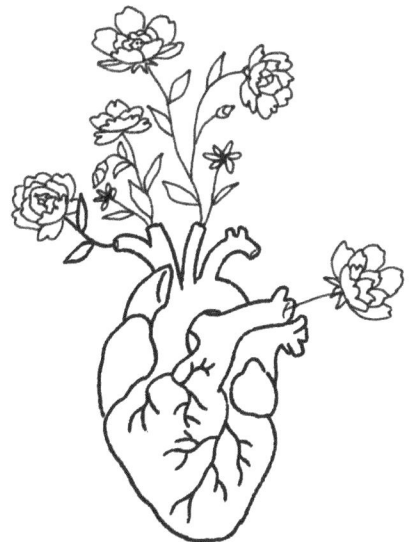

Stress

Science reveals that intense levels of stress damage the hippocampus, the part of the brain that remembers. That's why excess stress makes you forgetful. Doing too many activities at once—multitasking—diffuses attention, fatigues the brain, and adds stress. In contrast, physical exercise brings oxygen to the brain. Walking, dancing, and other movement activities create new pathways in the brain.

Stress and pain come into your life. Tissues become tender with inflammation. Inflammation is a byproduct of stress and leads to lower immunity.

Reducing stress increases your immunity and decreases inflammation. Doing the same thing over and over, you get what you've always gotten. If you want something different, try something new. Don't just pick up where you left off. See the new place you want to go. Create it.

Stress can overwhelm the nervous system, creating tension in the body and mind. It lowers your immunity, creating a ripe environment for some form of disease. Stress accumulates toxins in your body. Stress has its own biological markers, chemicals such as cortisol and cortisone. Functioning slows down. It becomes retarded, impaired. Breathe. Take the inhalation in through your nose. Exhale through your mouth and make a sound. Trauma

Here is the skinny on trauma and your body. Trauma is an experience or accumulated experiences that overwhelm the nervous system. Trauma in the context of this book is broad, including anything that overwhelms your nervous system, like chronic stress.

What is your trauma? Maybe it was not personal but generational. Multiple generations harboring the same secret, engaging in the same behavior, creating the same experience so it may finally be worked out. You are a byproduct of your ancestors. It is not just about being a pull-yourself-up-by-your-bootstraps rugged individual. Many physical patterns are genetic, generational, historical, hereditary, and/or environmental.

Trauma is psychological and physiological. Your body is an organic vessel. Experiences nurture your body, as do food, love, people, community.

The vagus nerve runs into the center of your being—your solar plexus. It comes through your body from your head/neck area. The parasympathetic nervous system joins with the polyvagal system, the vagus nerve, and creates nerve endings in the center of your being. You feel in your gut. You know in your gut. How often have you bypassed that gut feeling? That gut feeling is your body's way of sending you vital information. Bypass happens. You are in a rush, you didn't eat, didn't sleep enough, didn't notice. You missed the information.

Consider the fear you have lived with, the stress incurred and caused. Take a moment and recount your tale.

Triggers engage symptoms. Your neocortex is abandoned. Reptilian brain prevails; it is reflexive. You do what you have overlearned and integrated into your body, a kinesthetic memory. You stop breathing or breathe shallowly. Your heart races. You feel panic, anxiety. Run. Hide. Shrink. This is trauma amplified. You have micro-moments of this that are more common—discord in relationship, financial stress, and/or difficulties at work. These experiences may not overwhelm your nervous system individually, but together they accumulate and you feel it. Something is off. Your gut tells you. Listen to what it says. Note it here.

How has (fill in the blank) contributed to trauma in your life?

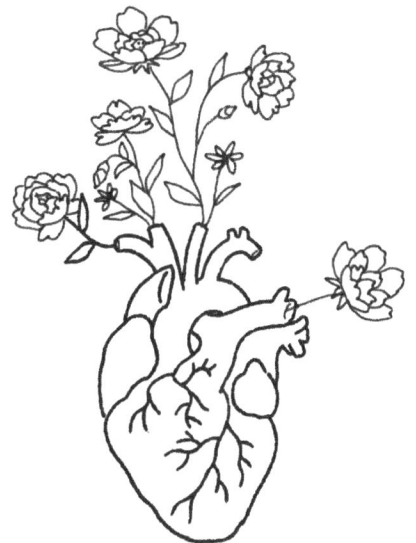

Rituals are profound demarcations of time and place. They are profound because they are imbued with meaning. They mark an emotion or let an emotion be expressed deeply to allow movement to the future, to allow release of the past. This is over. This will begin. You are here to support you and love you. This is part of the path of healing. A ritual of letting go. Of grieving the loss. This can be done with a shaman, a healer, a clergy, a sister, a friend, or by yourself. Allow a witness to be present. Allow them to follow your pain and acknowledge it. Heal and commemorate this moment. You are seen. You are not invisible.

More Farewells

This can be abstract, like who you used to be, your former self, before a life changing event. It can be more concrete, as a farewell to a relationship. Think about farewells you have attended—memorials, funerals, celebrations of life, remembrances of someone who touched you and/or your life. What can you extract from these experiences? What can you incorporate in our own ritual?

A prompt:

"Goodbye _____. You served me well. Gave me _____. Now what I want is_____."

Rituals are personal. They are created by you. These are suggestions, but not necessarily the forms you must adopt. What is most meaningful to you?

One ritual is to write yourself a letter about your pain, loss, grief, and then burn it. Allow it to go up in flames. Fire is purifying.

The letter identifies:

- What happened. Just the facts.

- How you felt about that experience.

- What you want yourself or another person to know.

Forgive yourself first. Explore that.

Forgive others when you are ready. If someone has hurt you, acknowledge their transgressions.

Do not minimize them. No need to overstate them. Just write the facts and how you felt about them. Once you are ready, write a letter of forgiveness. This letter is for you, not to you, but to them. This letter is for you to burn, to delete, to save. It is not to give to the other person, rarely is that necessary, except when it is and you'll know. If it is necessary, write a letter or have a conversation with them if you can, or do both. You'll know. Trust your gut. This is the process. You are doing it. Forgive yourself. You're doing fine.

Write an outline of the letter here.

Rewrite it on a separate sheet of paper.

Then burn it.

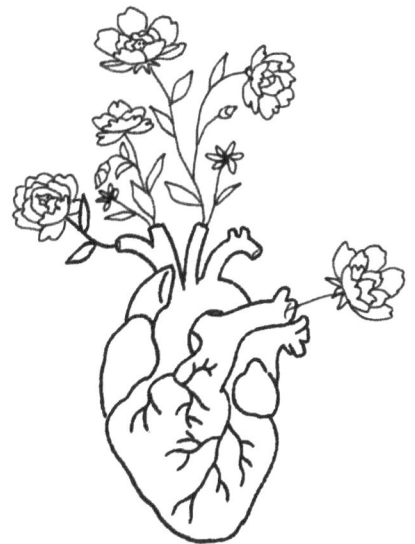

Another option is to use your voice. Shout out or wail your grief in the silence of the forest, your pillow, your car. Or allow others to witness it. Or do both. Read your letter aloud. Wail and be witnessed. There is power here.

Another ritual is to get a tattoo—henna, marker, applique. Often women have used body art to cover or incorporate scars—to glorify, dignify, or beautify their body where they once felt ugly, aging, unloved. Now it is love. These are suggestions. Try one or create your own.

Draw the image of your tattoo.

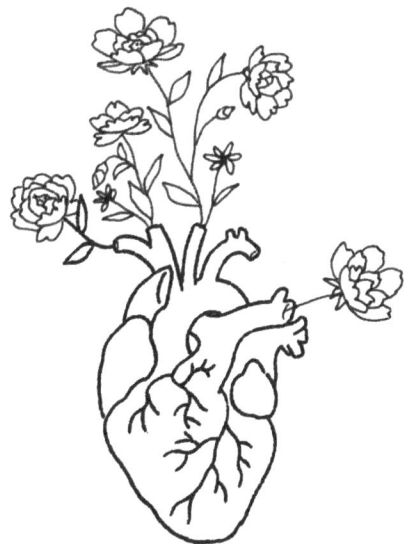

Be gentle.

I forgive myself for _____.

I forgive my body for _____.

I forgive my mind for _____.

I forgive _____.

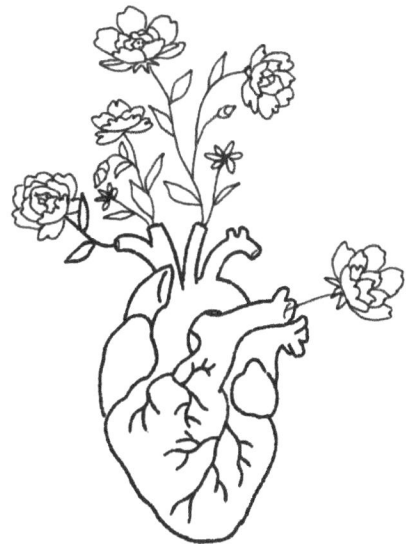

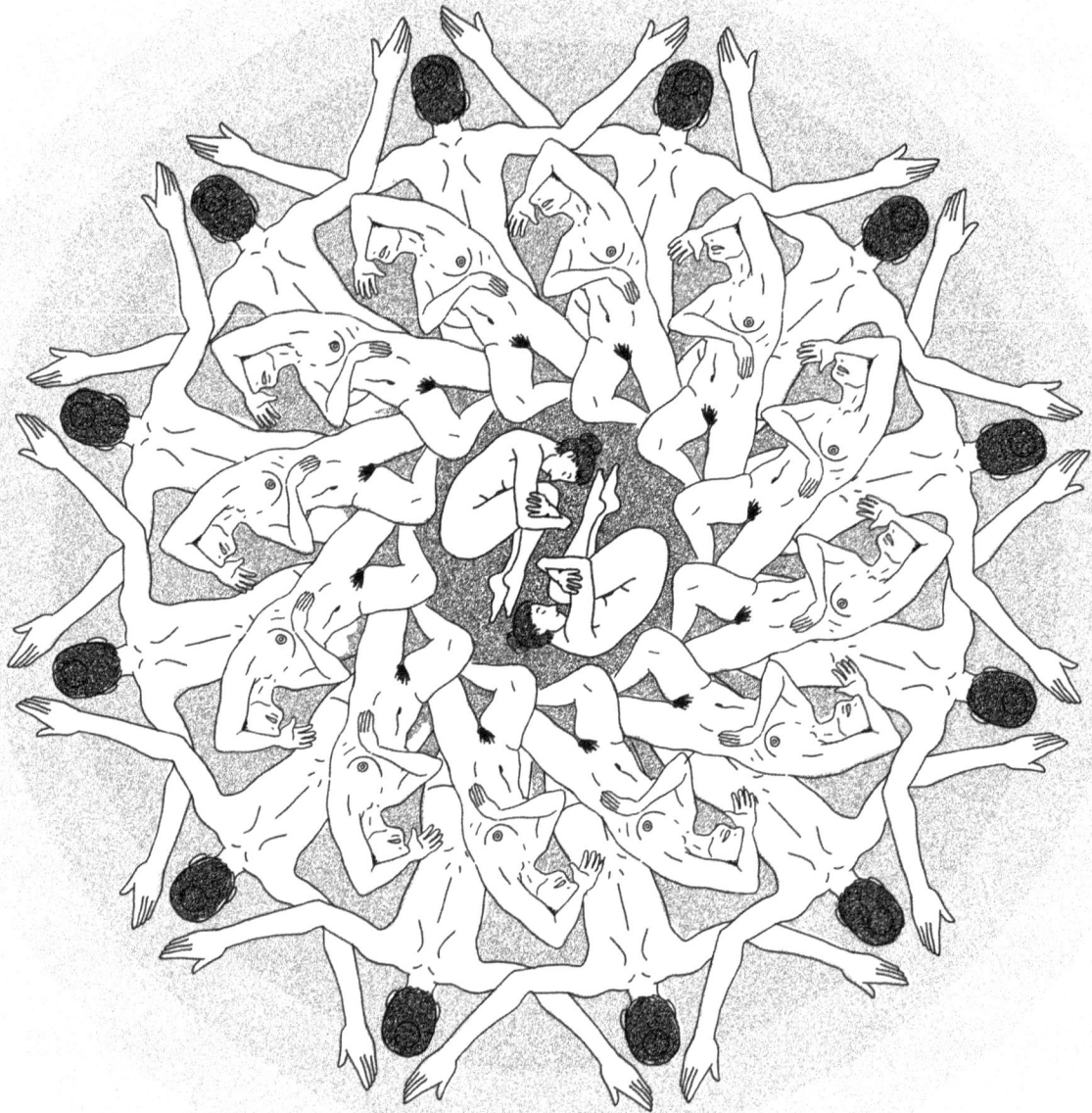

Understanding Women's Sexual Response Cycle

"The idea of synchronizing her outer movements with the natural rhythms

of her body inspired her."

—*Tami Lynn Kent, Wild Feminine*

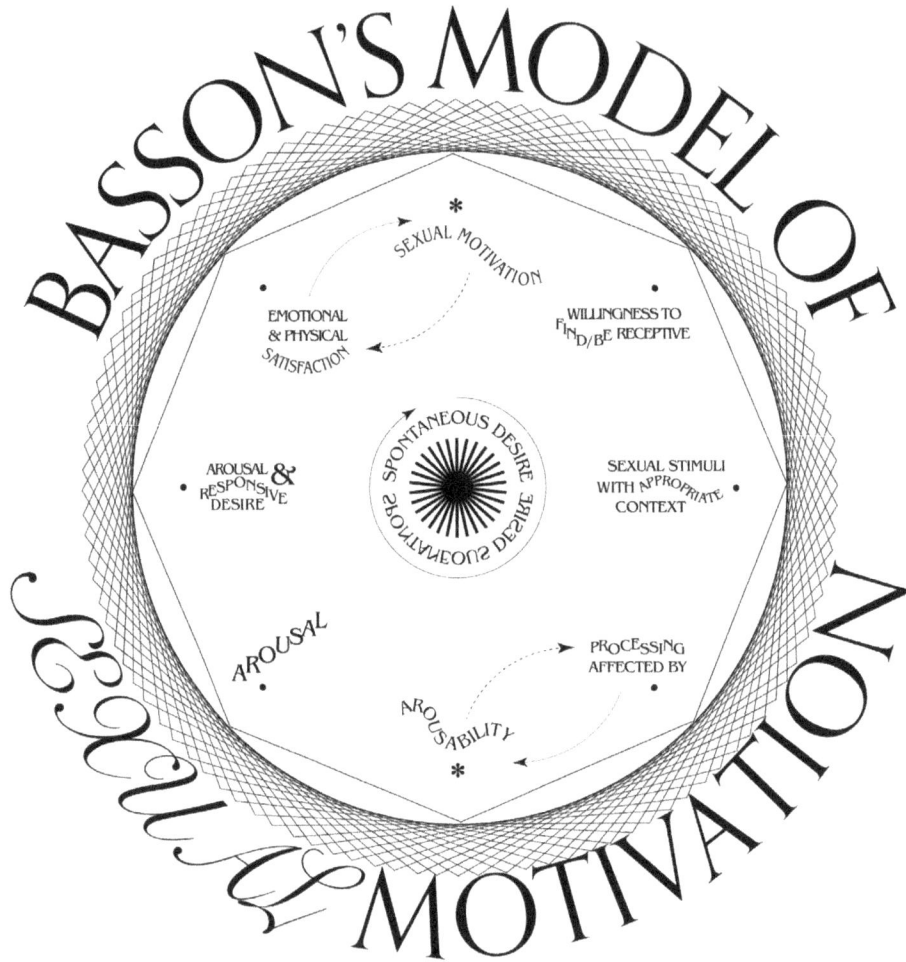

BASSON'S MODEL OF SEXUAL MOTIVATION

SEXUAL MOTIVATION

EMOTIONAL & PHYSICAL SATISFACTION

WILLINGNESS TO FIND/BE RECEPTIVE

SPONTANEOUS DESIRE
SPONTANEOUS DESIRE

AROUSAL & RESPONSIVE DESIRE

SEXUAL STIMULI WITH APPROPRIATE CONTEXT

AROUSAL

PROCESSING AFFECTED BY

AROUSABILITY

Female Sexual Response cycle by Basson

The duration of each phase and the intensity of the experience may vary for you and be different every time

you are aroused.

The sexual response cycle refers to the physical and emotional changes that occur when you are aroused sexually. Knowing how your body may respond during each phase increases your knowledge of sexuality, your understanding of your unique response, and your confidence about being sexual. Women are complex and dynamic: we have more nerve endings, more complexity for orgasm, more erogenous zones.

Sexual Arousal

Women don't always experience excitement first. Arousal may beget desire. This stage of arousal may last a few minutes to several hours. Physiological symptoms include but are not limited to: increased heart rate, blood flow, muscle tension, vaginal lubrication, and breathing; as well as swelling of the clitoris, labia minora, vaginal walls, breasts, etc.

What does sexual arousal look like for you? What does it feel like?

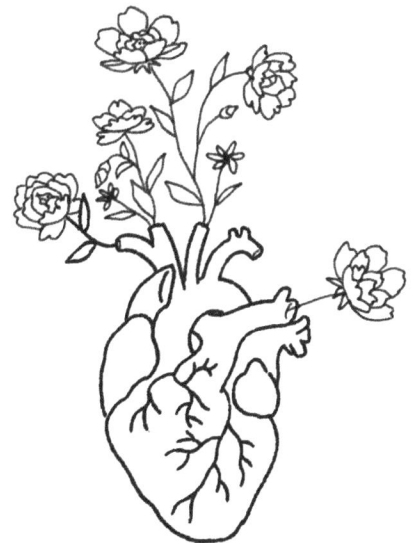

Arousal & Sexual Desire

In this phase, the above characteristics are intensified until you are at the edge of orgasm. The clitoris becomes highly sensitive and may retract. Muscle tension may become muscle spasms in the body.

What is it like to focus on your arousal and desire? Can you go there?

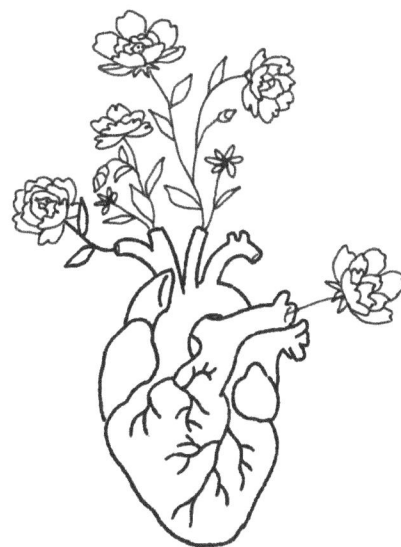

Emotional & Physical Satisfaction

This is the shortest phase, lasting a few seconds. However, for many, it is the most impactful.

There is further intensification of the above characteristics. You may notice a strong contraction

of muscles. This is involuntary, meaning you have no control over it. Contractions may be felt

in both the uterus and the vagina. A "sex flush" or redness may appear over the entire body.

Thinking about satisfaction, complete this prompt:

I remember _____.

I remember _____.

I remember _____.

Keep going.

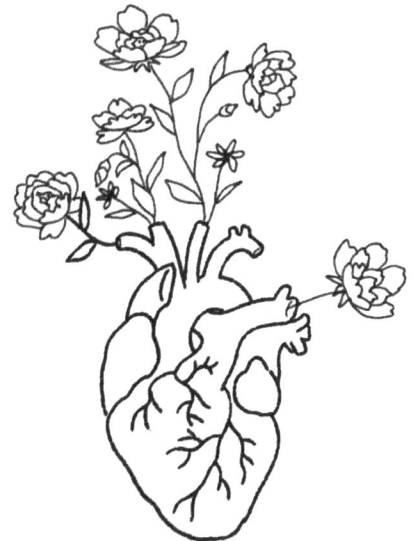

Emotional Intimacy

During this final phase, the body returns to its homeostasis. Mood may be elevated. Connection

to your partner(s) may be increased. This phase may easily lead to the sexual stimuli phase.

How does this work for you?

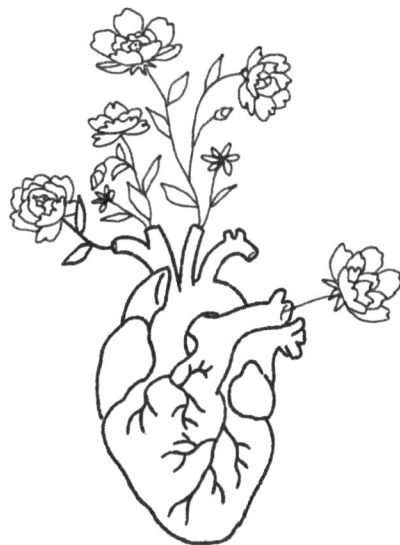

Sexual Stimuli

What turns you on? Draw your sexual stimuli here. List them.

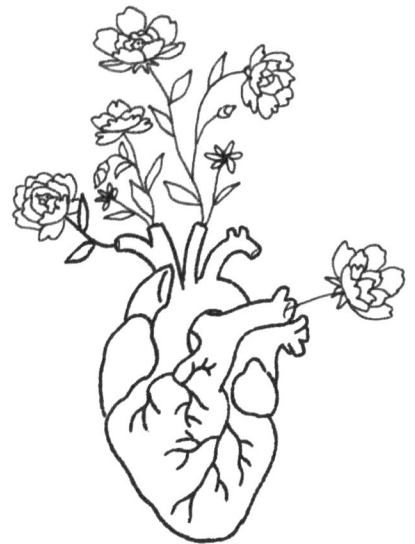

Take an afternoon or an hour or two to be with yourself. Play some music. Dance. Lie in the sun. Prepare and eat a delicious meal—your favorite. What does it take to turn you on? Not in a sexual way, but to turn you on so you feel fully alive. Take this time and explore.

Put flowers in your room. Uplift your spirit. Spray lavender. Lavender is a natural antimicrobial. It can make you feel cooler and cleaner after sweating.

Use your fingertips on the places of your body that you have banished. Imagine your internal parts: your colon, your ovaries, your uterus, etc. Acknowledge all that you were, all that you are, and all that you will become. It is time for change. You have changed. You have overcome all in mind, body, and spirit. Your body holds the stories of what you have endured. Share one here.

Feeling Sexy

First off, you know that sexy is in the brain. When you feel sexy, you are sexy. When you are confident, you show it and others know it. When you allow yourself to think sexy, you can be. Adjust the lighting in your bedroom. Everyone looks better by candlelight. This is a start. No lights, no problem. Wear a negligee that covers what you don't feel good about on your body. Camouflage. Begin to feel better. Instead of being numb or avoiding—whether you are avoiding pain or pleasure—accept it. Embrace it.

"Pain is not a punishment. Pleasure is not a reward."

—Pema Chodron.

Life happens. Accept what is so you may change and grow.

Present Moment

Observe the sensations of the body. Following the breath helps you come into the present moment. It is only in the present moment that your body can dwell. It is never in the future. It is never in the past. It is only here, in the now. How lovely! The breath is a vehicle to bring your mind into now. When your mind races, you may be thinking of the future.

What are your current thoughts? Future thinking creates anxiety. Past thinking creates depression. "How could I have done that?" "Why did that happen?" "What could I have done differently?" Past thinking, worries, and fears reinforce that which you cannot change. This perpetuates a cycle of hopelessness and powerlessness. This blocks you. This is how depression is.

Resist it by coming into the now. The now is where the body resides. The now is accessible through breath. Notice that it is difficult to stay here. Thoughts emerge. Then those thoughts pass. Noticing the sensations of the body can bring one into the present moment. Observe and be with them. Be with bodily sensations, like an orgasm. Work with sensations without getting attached, like to an orgasm. Orgasms come and orgasms go. Pain is the same. You may prefer the orgasm. It is okay to have a preference. That is part of who you are. Observe that you have a preference. Then let it go. Breathe. Exhale. Getting used to this? Observe the exhalation. Notice the preference. Become attuned to what is. Accept. Relax. Relaxation is critical for megawatt sex.

Maybe this is innocuous. Maybe it is completely triggering. That is okay. You are here with you. Feel the ridges with your fingers. Feel the numbness. Feel the pain of what was. Memory or sensation? Explore your body and your sensations. Allow them to exist. Allow them to come to your attention. The part of you that you usually ignore has come into focus. Focus with lightness. Focus and relax into it.

Desire & Hormonal Changes

Many factors can lower your sexual desire, including hormone treatments. Premenopause, estrogen comes directly from the ovaries. Postmenopause, estrogen, along with androgen, comes from the adrenal glands, which sit on top of the kidneys. These hormones directly impact your interest in sex. Postmenopausal women's process of losing their fertility is gradual. For some, fertility loss can be shockingly rapid.

Vaginal dryness, fatigue, mood changes, pain, and loss of confidence are symptoms that can impact sexual desire. Take time to understand your sexual desire. Do not rush things. Consider what your body needs.

Do you need more rest? How do you feel about how you look?

What is your energy level?

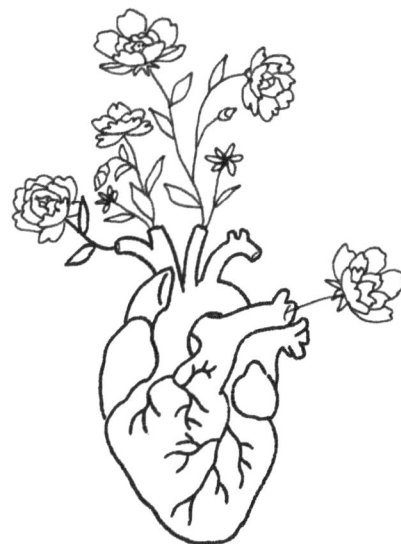

Vaginal Symptoms

Vaginal dryness is uncomfortable at best. It can increase the likelihood of vaginal infections.

Vaginal dryness and/or tightness may also result in pain during sex and decrease your ability to have an orgasm.

Vaginas dry with age. Pelvic radiation therapy can also narrow and shorten the vagina. It can decrease its elasticity, disrupt blood flow, and obstruct sexual response, possibly derailing your sexual self-image.

Estrogen

Estrogen rebuilds the lining of the vagina and the urethra, promotes collagen production, and helps maintain muscle tone. Phytoestrogens are plant-based estrogens found in plants such as black cohosh, evening primrose, and don quai. Applied locally in a low dose, estrogen can help mitigate some symptoms. Tablets are another option. Consult with your physician about hormone therapy and how estrogen might be used.

Dilators

Self-pleasure with the use of dilators and vaginal moisturizers or lubricants can help reduce symptoms such as vaginal pain, dryness, thinning tissue, inflammation, scar tissue, and shrinking/tightness. These symptoms impact the ability to achieve a satisfying orgasm, making it less intense or fulfilling.

Lubricants

Lubricants reduce friction and increase penetrability. There are three different types of lubricants, or lubes: water-based, silicone, and oil-based.

Water-based lubricants may dry out and become sticky and tacky. Saliva helps water-based lubricants stay slippery. They dissolve in water, so use a different lube in the hot tub.

Silicone does not evaporate, nor is it absorbed into the skin like a water-based lubricant. The feel is different, smoother. Silicone on silicone disintegrates. Don't use silicone lubricants on silicone toys. In addition to melting, it will allow bacterial growth.

Oil-based lubricants are either petroleum-based or food-grade. Almond oil, a food-grade oil, replenishes the female genitalia. It helps mitigate some of the above symptoms, such as pain.

Coconut oil is antimicrobial and antifungal. These oils are best used in their purest states. No added scents or flavors. Buy organic if you can. Remember—you are using this on sensitive areas.

Try placing either oil in your vagina overnight. Insert about 3 tablespoons of oil with a dropper or syringe. Use a towel as the oil may leak. See what happens. Do this for a week. Then insert dilators for 3 weeks before coitus. This is a vaginal rejuvenative and replenishes moisture.

Hot Flashes & Night Sweats

Hot flashes and night sweats are a buzzkill and, in general, can be difficult to live with. The good news is that they are an indicator that your metabolism is working.

The following suggestions can help reduce the frequency or duration of hot flashes and night sweats.

- Reduce your intake of coffee, tea, alcohol, sugar, and nicotine—really all the fun mood-altering drugs. If you can take them out of your life completely, you are a rock star!

- Keep your environment cool. Sip cool, refreshing drinks, like mint tea. Open windows. Allow a breeze. Lower the heat. Have some ventilation. Use a fan. Spray your face with an atomizer. Keep it by your bed and use it at night; rose is a cooling variety.

- Wear natural fiber clothing, like cotton or silk, that allows your body to breath. Avoid synthetic clothing. Sleep naked. Take off layers or covers. Shower before you sleep. Put a towel on your bed if you sweat a lot.

- Change the bed sheets before you get intimate with yourself or anyone else. Uplift the environment. Put an ice pack in your bed. That's cool. Just don't put it on your partner. It may not stop the hot flashes or sweating, but it limits the impact on you.

What helps?

Neuroplasticity & the Brain

Neuroplasticity is the ability of the brain to create new patterns of awareness out of existing patterns because the former ones are gone. The brain is forging a new path to experience or do a task that you could easily do using existing pathways. Neuroplasticity is important. It is here that you can create new erogenous zones, new ways of knowing love.

The first step is exploration of self. You are mind, body, spirit. Existing together. This numbness you feel may allow for new erogenous zones. It may allow for neuroplasticity. The brain can reorganize, adjust, and compensate.

Make new neural connections and create new erogenous zones by stimulating the skin. An important piece of enlivening the nerve endings is therapeutic touch. Touch that is healing and gentle. Touch that allows energy to flow into the body. Touch that increases circulation and limits scar tissue. Touch can invigorate health. Feel the pulse of life. Touch your sex organs. Fingertips, ears, and lips are erogenous zones.

The mind is the most important sex organ. Sexy is a state of mind. When a woman knows that, she can choose to act sexy, dress sexy, or behave in a sexy manner. Others will perceive her as sexy.

Choose increased intimacy. Be in the present moment and stay in relationship with yourself. This relies on a foundation of self-love and nurturance. Focus on that first. Please yourself delightfully. Hone that ability to create what you want. Believe it. Embrace all you love about yourself.

How do you currently embrace sexy?

How do you foster a sex-positive mindset

knowing that you experience sexual pleasure?

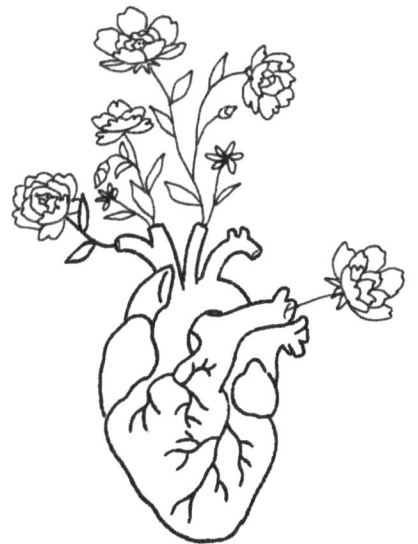

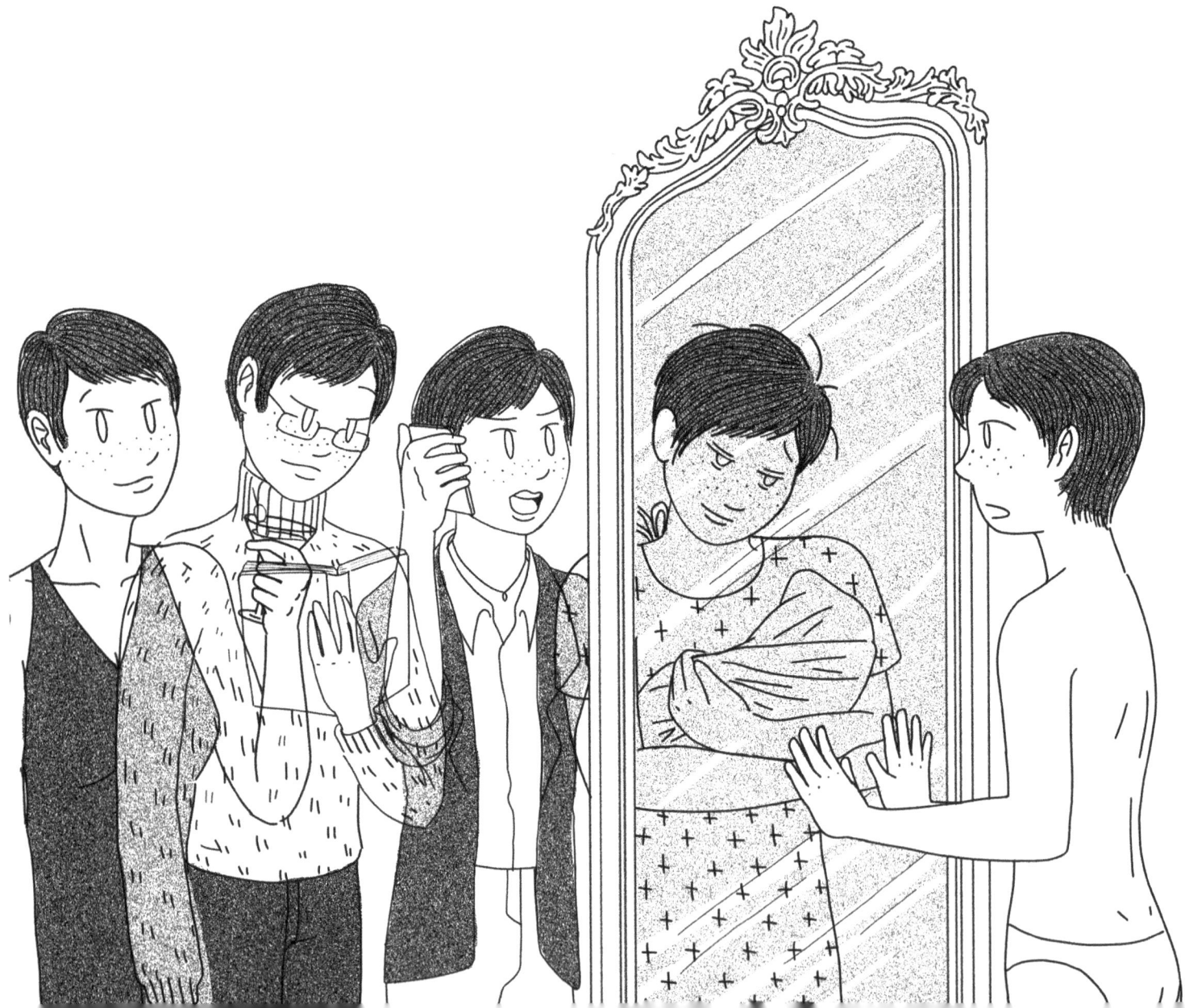

Reflecting on You

" She was becoming herself and daily casting aside that fictitious self which

we assume like a garment with which to appear before the world. "

—Kate Chopin, The Awakening

Congratulations

Celebrate yourself as a woman. Behold the miracle of your body, to be, to yield. Behold your glory. You are a goddess. You are a warrior within. Love your body. Love your body image. Round. Short. Fat. Tall. Thin. Mild. Meek. Loud. Warts. Freckles. Moles. Love handles. Behold. Cellulite. Love you. You are glorious. You are microcosms of life, too numerous to count. Infinitesimal organisms, bacteria, microbiomes living within you. With you. Creating life continuously. Behold. You are a miracle that you barely comprehend.

You have just done a whole lot of personal exploration. Congratulations. Remember what you've done. Honor it. You are fearless and brave.

Now that you have begun this journey, how will you continue?

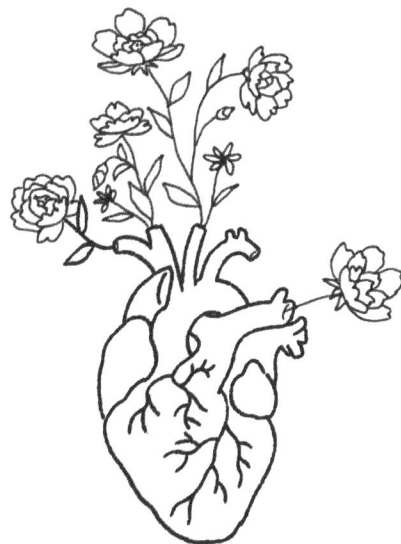

Review. Revisit. Rediscover the mysteries of you. Again. Celebrate all that you have learned and unlearned.

Sometimes you may want to revisit these journal pages and read them over. Other times you may want to rip them out and burn them, releasing them into the ethos. What do you choose?

Burn some pages.

Fire transforms.

Some pages
you may want to
crumple up and
throw away

to erase shame or
guilt about what
that page holds.

Note old patterns coming back and dictating behaviors. Release them.

Try something new. Review it. Release it. Build knowledge based on compassion for self.

Turn a page into poetry, lyrics, dance, song.

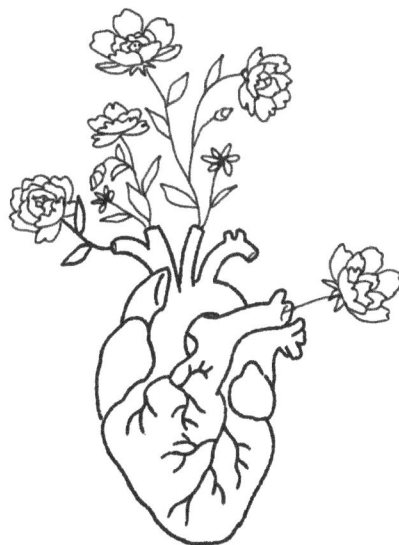

End this time and continue to discover more about you.

Practice gratitude for you—all you are and all you are becoming.

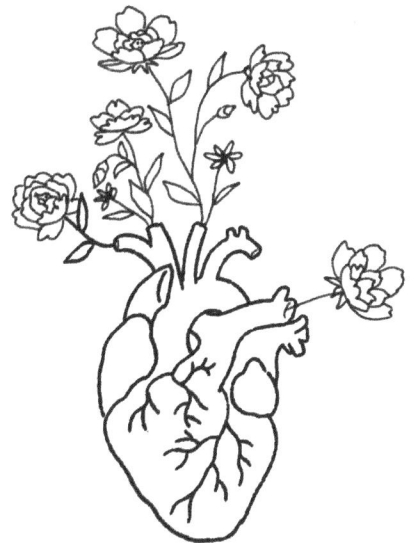

Family History

What have you received from your ancestors?

Is there a history or recurring pattern of (fill in the blank)?

Is that history true for you?

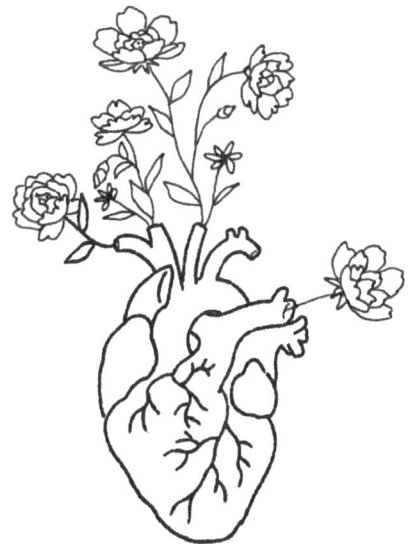

What Have You Learned?

Understanding how your engagement with this guidebook has impacted you is important. You have put yourself first, making a commitment to you, making time for your relationship with you. Continue to take the time. Schedule an appointment with yourself. Make it a priority. You deserve this. Now act on it.

How have you taken this on?

How will you proceed from here?

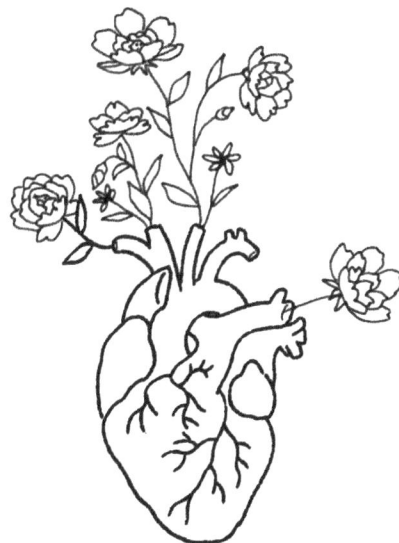

Take a day to read through your journal. Appreciate yourself. You did this for you.

Now, what is the next great thing that you will do for you?

List it here and beyond.

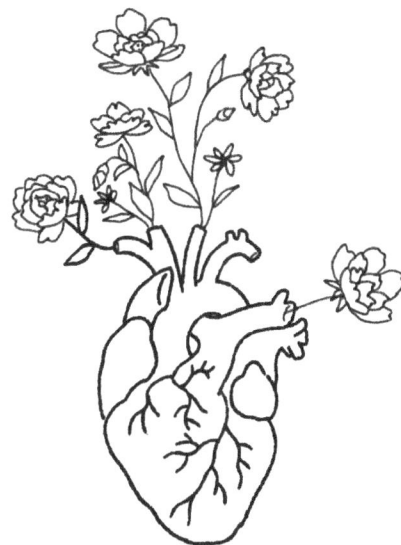

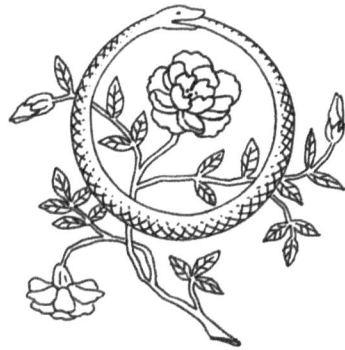

References

Brizendine, L. (2007). The Female Brain. Harmony.

Brown, B. (2019, August 22). Shame v. guilt. Brené Brown. https://brenebrown.com/blog/2013/01/14/shame-v-guilt/

Chopin, K. (2019). The Awakening. Independently published.

Flannery, J. A. (2017, November 3). What Basson's Sexual Response Cycle Teaches Us About Sexuality. Lifeworks Psychotherapy. https://www.lifeworkspsychotherapy.com/bassons-sexual-response-cycle-teaches-us-sexuality/#:%7E:text=Rosemary%20Basson%20would%20like%20us,women%20in%20long%2Dterm%20relationships.

Graham, M. (1991). Blood Memory. Washington Square.

Kent, T. L. (2011). Wild Feminine: Finding Power, Spirit & Joy in the Female Body (1st ed.). Atria Books/Beyond Words.

Lorde, A. (1984). Sister Outsider: Essays and Speeches, Crossing Press. Crossing Press.

Mani, M. (2020, May 12). This Maya Angelou Quote On Butterflies Will Inspire And Uplift You. Out of Stress. https://www.outofstress.com/we-delight-in-the-beauty-of-the-butterfly-maya-angelou-quote/

Mencimer, S. (2002, June 1). The trouble with Frida Kahlo: uncomfortable truths about this season's hottest female artist. Washington Monthly. https://washingtonmonthly.com/2001/06/01/the-trouble-with-frida-kahlo/

Meyer, H. (2014). Divine Path to Healing. Independently Published.

Monroe, V. (2001, October). Are Your Insecurities Ruining Your Sex Life? O, The Oprah Magazine. http://www.oprah.com/relationships/self-consciousness-during-sex-improving-body-image/all

Pain is not a punishment. Pleasure is not a reward. (2010, November 4). Mindfulness 4 Stress Reduction. https://mindfulness4stressreduction.com/2010/11/04/pain-pleasure

Bio

Tara Galeano is a certified sex therapist who has worked with women for over two decades to get their sexy back. She knows that there is pleasure in the body, beyond our wildest dreams, and every woman can access it. In Rediscovering My Body, Tara teaches women how to show up for pleasure in their lives. She rediscovered her own body after leaving her twenty-five-year marriage. Realizing that she had given so much of herself away, she knew that she needed to come back to the inherent wisdom of the body. Through reconnecting with her body, Tara was able to know what was true for her, how best to proceed from this wisdom, what was true pleasure, and most importantly, how to teach these lessons to other women who are clamoring for the same truths so that they too can transform their lives and reclaim their sensuality. Now Tara has embodied this path and is moving forward to share this with women everywhere with her book, her online courses and community, and her retreats. She lives in San Francisco with her soul sister and is learning how to live more fully in her nomadic heart.

www.ingramcontent.com/pod-product-compliance
Lightning Source LLC
Chambersburg PA
CBHW080557030426
42336CB00019B/3217